Clinical Nutrition, COVID-19, and Long COVID

(+ Vaccines, Graphene Oxide, Masks, and Other Viruses)

Holistic, Scientific, Natural, Herbal, Nature-Based Immunity and Recovery

Collin Gow, C.N.C.

Table of Contents

DISCLAIMER:

The contents of this book are not an attempt to treat, diagnose, prevent, or cure any disease or condition. Talk to your doctor before making any changes.

Immunity

Collin Gow, C.N.C.

1/28/2020

Supplements

Daily use:

Mushrooms (maitake, shiitake, chaga, reishi, cordyceps, agarikon...) - immunomodulators (immune balancers), antitumor, antiinflammatory, antiviral. Agarikon is the strongest antiviral known.

Andrographis - antiinflammatory, antiviral, antimicrobial, antiprotozoa, antioxidant, blood sugar.

Astragalus - immunomodulator, anti-aging, adrenal health, kidney health, energy.

Echinacea (full spectrum extract) - boosts white blood cells including natural killer cells, moves and cleanses lymph. Good for pain in the neck under the jaw from swollen lymph nodes.

Olive leaf - contains oleuropein. Antifungal, antiviral, antibacterial, heart health, blood pressure, blood sugar. Slows viral shedding, budding, assembly, and replication.

Cat's Claw - antiinflammatory, immunodulator, antioxidant, antihypertensive, increases phagocytosis.

Licorice, marshmallow, aloe, slippery elm - immune cell communication, inhibit antigens of pathogens from attaching to cells, antiviral. Good for dry coughs and sore throats.

Aged garlic extract - immunomodulator, anticarcinogenic, Th1 immune responses, antioxidant.

Plant sterols - immunomodulators, do not take if you have very low cholesterol levels.

Elderberry - antiviral, febrifuge (lowers fever), decongestant. Good choice for kids because it tastes good.

Prebiotics, Probiotics, Postbiotics - 70% of the immune system is in the gut and there's more bacteria in your body than there are cells. Probiotics are foundational for a myriad of immune responses.

Shilajit/humic & fulvic acid - antiviral, immunomodulator, pro & anti-inflammatory, GABA mimetic.

Lysine - blocks the receptor sites where viruses try to secrete enzymes to spread through the body.

Vitamin A, C, E, D3, Zinc, Selenium - foundational vitamins and minerals which provide a host of immune benefits - NK cells, neutrophils, innate & adaptive immunity, macrophages, T & B cells, etc.

Colostrum or IGG - good source of antibodies. Antibodies tag pathogens so your immune system knows to destroy them. Important for innate immunity, GI health, and non-breastfed adults & children.

Temporary use:

Goldenseal - contains berberine. Antibacterial, anti-fungal, anti-protozoa, anti-viral, blood sugar, heart health, anti-inflammatory, anti-tumor. Good for pain in neck under the jaw line due to swollen lymph.

Grapefruit seed extract - antibacterial, antifungal, antiprotozoa, antiviral.

Silver - antiviral, antifungal, antibacterial, antiprotozoa. Good for ear, nose, throat, and eye infections.

Oregano oil - contains carvacrol. Antifungal, antibacterial, antiviral, antiprotozoa. Good for sinus congestion and respiratory infections in general.

Garlic containing allicin - antimicrobial, antifungal, antiviral, antiinflammatory.

Foods/Lifestyle

Limit processed foods and refined sugars. Limit high arginine foods (chocolate and nuts). Limit iron intake from foods and supplements. **Limit dairy, meat, and other animal foods (organ meats are ok). Eat mushrooms, garlic, onions, ginger, peppers, fermented foods, manuka honey, citrus fruits, seaweed, and nutritional yeast. Nasal sprays, essential oils such as the four thieves remedy, ear oils, and hand washing** are other precautionary measures one can take to reduce the spread of germs.

Coronavirus 101

Collin Gow, C.N.C.
2/28/20

Dear loyal clients, friends, and family,

This **flu season** has been an especially anxious and distressing one, with the **Coronavirus** threatening to become a pandemic. It's important not to panic, yet it is also important to take the necessary precautions to protect you and your loved ones. I have you and your family in my thoughts during this time and I am ready at the helm with natural remedies and immune system boosters to bolster your defenses. I thought I should prepare a short briefing on this topic and list my **top 10 recommended supplements** for your immune system.

What you need to know:

- Coronavirus was first detected in Wuhan City, Hubei Province, China and has now been detected in 57 locations internationally, including in the United States.
- It is a new form of the virus and it allegedly originated from bats.
- It causes respiratory disease and may cause death.
- It has been declared a public health emergency of international concern by the WHO.
- While cases have been detected in the U.S., according to the CDC, as of 2/28/20, the virus is NOT currently spreading in the community in the U.S.
- It spreads via animal to person and/or person to person via coughing, sneezing, close contact, etc. and can spread before a person has any symptoms.

My Top 10 Supplements

1. Astragalus
2. Silver
3. Oregano Oil
4. Olive Leaf
5. Vitamins A, C, D, E, Zinc, and Selenium
6. Elderberry
7. Andrographis
8. Mushrooms (Fomitopsis officinalis, Reishi, Shiitake, Maitake, Turkey Tail, Cordyceps, Chaga, etc.)
9. Echinacea
10. Berberine or Goldenseal

Other great options:

Pre, pro, and postbiotics, shilajit, colostrum or IGG, cat's claw, licorice or marshmallow, mucolase, oscillococcinum, garlic, grapefruit seed extract, lomatium, NAC, pleurisy, horehound, mullein, elecampane, yerba santa, thyme, eucalyptus, wild cherry bark, black seed oil, lysine, burdock.

What else?

Limit processed foods and refined sugars. Limit high arginine foods (chocolate and nuts). Limit iron intake from foods and supplements. Limit dairy, meat, and other animal foods. Eat mushrooms, garlic, onions, ginger, peppers, fermented foods, manuka honey, citrus fruits, seaweed, coconut, Brazil nuts, & nutritional yeast. Nasal sprays, essential oils, ear oils, and hand washing are also precautionary measures one can take which may possibly reduce the spread of germs. Should you come down with any virus this season, I recommend taking A LOT more than the bottle recommends just to be safe! Tripling, quadrupling, quintupling, or sextupling the recommended doses may be necessary! Ask your doctor or email me, however, and I/we will guide you on this. If you are a confirmed carrier of the Coronavirus, **seek immediate medical attention** and take measures so as not to spread the virus to others. In gratitude for your continued support of me, I am here to support you. Stay safe and be well.

Pandemic 101

Collin Gow, C.N.C.
2/29/20

Dear citizens,

This **pandemic season** as of 2/29/20 has been an especially anxious and distressing one, as it usually is. The pattern continues, whether it's **swine flu, bird flu, SARS, MERS, west nile, ebola, zika, coronavirus**, or others, it seems that almost every year there's a new pathogen poised to reach pandemic proportions. Could any of these microbes have been perpetrated on the masses purposely to strike fear and obedience into them? It seems possible, if not likely, given such a predictable **pattern**. Out comes the virus, of which a patent on the vaccine for it was filed a year prior in secrecy, then it spreads, then ensues mass hysteria, it's all over every news channel, the experts warned of it a few months back, soon there's talk of a vaccine, then we are all saved by the mighty cow gods, then it mysteriously vanishes into thin air and we never think of it again (probably because there's another one next year to entertain us and draw our attention away from more important issues). The plan always seems to play out perfectly for the pharmaceutical companies and their pundits like precision clockwork. If indeed they are behind the farce, that is. The profits pour in while the poor press on, ignorant to the scheme of the billionaires. It matters little, however. You are likely not a billionaire and you must deal with the vermin that has been unleashed that threatens to vanquish you this very minute. It's important not to panic in this time of uncertainty and chaos, while the death toll allegedly rises, yet it is also important to take the necessary precautions to protect you and your loved ones. No, I don't mean using hand sanitizer and water and antibacterial soap. These are useful, sure, but I'm talking about real precautions. I do believe people are dying and I do believe the pathogen is real. So, I'm ready at the helm with natural remedies and immune system boosters to bolster your defenses. Your immune system is what you need most right now. So, here's a short briefing on this topic and my **top 10 natural antivirals/antimicrobials and immune system strengtheners**. Call it **Natural Pandemic Preparedness 101**, plus, some food recommendations to boot. I know, I know, I went way too far off the deep end on this one.

What to do when a pandemic strikes:

- Distrust the mainstream media (6 corporations own all of the mainstream media outlets)
- Do your own research
- Take it in perspective/proportion/context (realize that many more people die from the food they put in their mouths and from cancer and heart disease than any pathogen will probably ever cause. The media likes to blow things out of proportion to other important stories to push its agenda)
- Prepare yourself regardless (don't get so wrapped up in conspiracies about this year's pandemic that you don't take precautionary measures to protect and prepare yourself)
- Eat healthily
- Buy a face mask
- Stock up on natural medicines

My Top 10 Supplements

1. Astragalus
2. Silver
3. Oregano Oil
4. Olive Leaf
5. Vitamins A, C, D, E, Zinc, and Selenium

6. Elderberry
7. Andrographis
8. Mushrooms (Fomitopsis officinalis, Reishi, Shiitake, Maitake, Turkey Tail, Cordyceps, Chaga, etc.)
9. Echinacea
10. Berberine/Goldenseal

Other great options:
Pre, pro, and postbiotics, shilajit, colostrum or IGG, cat's claw, licorice or marshmallow, mucolase, oscillococcinum, garlic, grapefruit seed extract, lomatium, NAC, pleurisy, horehound, mullein, elecampane, yerba santa, thyme, eucalyptus, wild cherry bark, black seed oil, lysine, burdock.

What else?
Limit processed foods and refined sugars. Limit high arginine foods (chocolate and nuts). Limit iron intake from foods and supplements. Limit dairy, meat, and other animal foods. Eat mushrooms, garlic, onions, ginger, peppers, fermented foods, manuka honey, citrus fruits, seaweed, coconut, Brazil nuts, & nutritional yeast. Nasal sprays, essential oils, ear oils, and hand washing are also precautionary measures one can take which may possibly reduce the spread of germs. Should you come down with any virus this season, I recommend taking A LOT more than the bottle recommends just to be safe! Tripling, quadrupling, quintupling, or sextupling the recommended doses may be necessary! Ask your doctor or email me, however, and I/we will guide you on this. If you are a confirmed carrier of the Coronavirus, **seek immediate medical attention** and take measures so as not to spread the virus to others. In gratitude for your continued support of me, I am here to support you. Stay safe and be well.

Compendium of Clinical Studies Demonstrating Efficacy of Natural Compounds Against Coronaviruses

by Collin Gow, C.N.C. (3/18/2020)

"Griffithsin, a Highly Potent Broad-Spectrum Antiviral Lectin from Red Algae: From Discovery to Clinical Application"

"**GRFT is a red algae-derived lectin** of 121 amino acids ([Figure 1](#)). It exhibits potent (EC50 in the picomolar range) and broad-spectrum antiviral activity and negligible in vitro and in vivo host toxicity [9]. Its antiviral activity relates to a unique structural feature that forms a homodimeric complex with three carbohydrate-binding domains on each monomer ([Figure 2](#)). These three carbohydrate-binding domains **target high-mannose arrays present on many pathogenic enveloped viruses including** HIV; severe, acute, or **Middle East respiratory syndrome coronaviruses (SARS-CoV or MERS-CoV)** [10,11]; hepatitis C virus (HCV) [12,13]; herpes simplex virus 2 (HSV-2) [14,15]; Japanese encephalitis virus (JEV) [16,17]; and porcine epidemic diarrhea virus (PEDV) [18]. As a result of its broad antiviral spectrum, it shows great promise as a general microbicidal agent that can prevent viral transmission and as a therapeutic against enveloped virus-mediated diseases."

Lee, C. Griffithsin, a Highly Potent Broad-Spectrum Antiviral Lectin from Red Algae: From Discovery to Clinical Application. *Mar. Drugs* **2019**, *17*, 567.

"Antiviral Natural Products and Herbal Medicines"

"There are no specific treatments for CoV infection and preventive vaccines are still being explored. Thus, the situation reflects the need to develop effective antivirals for prophylaxis and treatment of CoV infection. We have previously reported that saikosaponins (A, B2, C, and D), which are **naturally** occurring triterpene glycosides isolated from medicinal plants such as *Bupleurum* spp. (柴胡 Chái Hú), *Heteromorpha* spp., and *Scrophularia scorodonia* (玄參 Xuán Shēn), exert antiviral activity against HCoV-22E9.[14] Upon co-challenge with the virus, these natural compounds effectively prevent the early stage of HCoV-22E9 infection, including viral attachment and penetration. Extracts from *Lycoris radiata* (石蒜 Shí Suàn), *Artemisia annua* (黃花蒿 Huáng Huā Hāo), *Pyrrosia lingua* (石葦 Shí Wěi), and *Lindera aggregata* (烏藥 Wū Yào) have also been documented to display **anti–SARS-CoV effect** from a screening analysis using hundreds of Chinese medicinal herbs.[15] Natural inhibitors against the SARS-CoV enzymes, such as the nsP13 helicase and 3CL protease, have been identified as well and include myricetin, scutellarein, and phenolic compounds from *Isatis indigotica* (板藍根 Bǎn Lán Gēn) and *Torreya nucifera* (榧 Fěi).[16,17,18] Other anti-CoV natural medicines include the water extract from *Houttuynia cordata* (魚腥草 Yú Xīng Cǎo), which has been observed to exhibit several antiviral mechanisms against SARS-CoV, such as inhibiting the viral 3CL protease and blocking the viral RNA-dependent RNA polymerase activity.[19]"

Lin, Liang-Tzung et al. "Antiviral natural products and herbal medicines." *Journal of traditional and complementary medicine* vol. 4,1 (2014): 24-35. doi:10.4103/2225-4110.124335

"Glycyrrhizin, an active component of liquorice roots, and replication of SARS-associated coronavirus."

"We assessed the antiviral potential of ribavirin, 6-azauridine, pyrazofurin, mycophenolic acid, and glycyrrhizin against two clinical isolates of coronavirus (FFM-1 and FFM-2) from patients with SARS admitted to the clinical centre of Frankfurt University, Germany. **Of all the compounds, glycyrrhizin [licorice] was the most active in inhibiting replication of the SARS-associated virus. Our findings suggest that glycyrrhizin should be assessed for treatment of SARS.**"

Cinatl, J et al. "Glycyrrhizin, an active component of liquorice roots, and replication of SARS-associated coronavirus." *Lancet (London, England)* vol. 361,9374 (2003): 2045-6. doi:10.1016/s0140-6736(03)13615-x

"In vitro susceptibility of 10 clinical isolates of SARS coronavirus to selected antiviral compounds."

"**Commercial antiviral agents and pure chemical compounds extracted from traditional Chinese medicinal herbs were screened against 10 clinical isolates of SARS coronavirus by neutralisation tests with confirmation by plaque reduction assays.** Interferon-beta-1a, leukocytic interferon-alpha, ribavirin, lopinavir, rimantadine, **baicalin [Chinese skullcap] and glycyrrhizin [licorice] showed antiviral activity."**

Chen, F et al. "In vitro susceptibility of 10 clinical isolates of SARS coronavirus to selected antiviral compounds." *Journal of clinical virology : the official publication of the Pan American Society for Clinical Virology* vol. 31,1 (2004): 69-75. doi:10.1016/j.jcv.2004.03.003

"Small molecules targeting severe acute respiratory syndrome human coronavirus"

"Compounds 5 (Aescin, a drug widely used in Europe) and **13** (Reserpine, a Food and Drug Administration-approved drug) **were further tested** with IFA, ELISA, Western blot analysis, and flow cytometry to confirm their anti-SARS activities. The EC50 values for Reserpine (compound **13**) and Aescin (compound **5**) were 3.4 μM and 6.0 μM, respectively, and the corresponding CC50 values were 25 μM (SI = 7.3) and 15 μM (SI = 2.5).

Aescin, the major active principle from the horse chestnut tree, has previously been used to treat patients with chronic venous insufficiency ([30](#), [31](#)), hemorrhoids ([32](#)), postoperative edema ([30](#), [32](#)), and inflammatory action ([30](#), [33](#)). Reserpine, a naturally occurring alkaloid produced by several members of the genus Rauwolfia, has been used primarily as a peripheral antihypertensive and as a central depressant and sedative ([34](#)). It has also found use as a radio-protective agent and experimentally as a contraceptive ([35](#)).

Because Glycyrrhizin, Aescin [horse chestnut] and Reserpine **have been used clinically, their related natural products may be also active against SARS-CoV.** We used the International Species Information System (ISIS) database to search for commercially available compounds whose structures have 80% similarities with these three drugs. We found 15 compounds related to Glycyrrhizin and Aescin and six compounds related to Reserpine. Through a cell-based assay, **we found that 10 of the 21 compounds showed activities against SARS-CoV. Among them, four compounds (6, 16, 17, and 18) are derivatives of Glycyrrhizin and Aescin, and all six derivatives of Reserpine (19–24) showed activities toward SARS-CoV at <100 μM.**

Some other well known traditional Chinese herbs were also tested in the cell-based assay and most of them were found inactive **against SARS-CoV** at the concentration of 10 μM. However, **we found that extracts of eucalyptus and *Lonicera japonica* did show such activities at the concentration of 100 μM; and Ginsenoside-Rb1 (17), one of the pharmacologically active components of Panax ginseng** ([42](#), [43](#))

Finally, previous reports in the literature have predicted that several compounds may show antiviral activities against SARS, such as AG7088 ([21](#)), Pentoxifylline ([45](#)), **Melatonin ([46](#)), and Vitamin C ([47](#)). However, our cell-based assay showed that these compounds had no effects at the concentration of 10 μM.** Some other anti-RNA virus drugs, such as AZT, Didanosine, Nevirapine, Ritonavir, Lopinavir, Saquinavir, and Ribavirin, also showed no activities at the same concentration."

Wu, Chung-Yi et al. "Small molecules targeting severe acute respiratory syndrome human coronavirus." *Proceedings of the National Academy of Sciences of the United States of America* vol. 101,27 (2004): 10012-7. doi:10.1073/pnas.0403596101

"Identification of natural compounds with antiviral activities against SARS-associated coronavirus"

"After primary screening, active compounds were cherry picked and a second round of test was performed for their antiviral effects. The pictures were taken to record cell morphology change caused by CPE and the inhibition effects of the compounds before MTS assay. As shown in Fig. 1, **four of the extracts, Lycoris radiata, Artemisia annua, Pyrrosia lingua, and Lindera aggregata exhibited significant inhibition effects on virus-induced CPE when SARS-CoV strain BJ001 was used in screening.**
Out of the four, Lycoris radiata was most potent.
One of the active samples which showed better inhibition effect in anti-SARS-CoV screening, L. radiata extract, was chosen for further identification of the active component in it. We first isolated the total alkaloid from L. radiata according to previous reports (Hong and Ma, 1964). We then examined its antiviral activity. This was based on previous findings that the majority of bioactive components of L. radiata were from its alkaloid fraction (Takagi et al., 1968; Miyasaka and Hiramatsu, 1980; Cortese et al., 1983). **From CPE/MTS assays, the isolated alkaloid showed potent inhibitory activity against SARS-CoV infection"**

Li, Shi-You et al. "Identification of natural compounds with antiviral activities against SARS-associated coronavirus." *Antiviral research* vol. 67,1 (2005): 18-23. doi:10.1016/j.antiviral.2005.02.007

"Herbal plants and plant preparations as remedial approach for viral diseases"

"Dioscorea Extracts. Patent No. US 20090041803; Filed September 02, 2008 [106]

This extract is an immunogenic composition that contains an antigen agent and an adjuvant agent, wherein the adjuvant agent contains an extract that is prepared from a tuber of a Dioscorea plant. This extract is prepared from the tuber of any of these **Dioscorea species namely D. batatas, D. ecne, D. alata L., D. pseudojaponica, or D. alata L. var. purpurea.** The antigen agent can be a polypeptide, such as a viral protein or a tumor antigen protein or a nucleic acid encoding the polypeptide. The invention is useful in but not limited to treating viral diseases such as infection by an adenovirus, a herpesvirus (e.g., HSV-I, HSV-II, CMV, or VZV), a poxvirus (e.g., an orthopoxvirus such as variola or vaccinia, or molluscum contagiosum), a picornavirus (e.g., rhinovirus or enterovirus), an orthomyxovirus (e.g., influenzavirus), a paramyxovirus [e.g., parainfluenzavirus, mumps virus, measles virus, and respiratory syncytial virus (RSV)], **a coronavirus (e.g., SARS)**, a papovavirus (e.g., papillomaviruses, such as those that cause genital warts, common warts, or plantar warts), a hepadnavirus (e.g., hepatitis B virus), a flavivirus (e.g., hepatitis C virus or Dengue virus), or a retrovirus (e.g., a lentivirus such as HIV). This herbal preparation also can be used as a dietary supplement, health food, or health drink for prevention of immune system impairment. It also finds use in treating a range of bacterial, fungal and neoplastic diseases."

Ganjhu, Rajesh Kumar et al. "Herbal plants and plant preparations as remedial approach for viral diseases." *Virusdisease* vol. 26,4 (2015): 225-36. doi:10.1007/s13337-015-0276-6

"Potential antivirals and antiviral strategies against SARS coronavirus infections."

"**Various other compounds**, often with an ill-defined mode of action but selectivity indexes up to 100, **have been reported to exhibit** *in vitro* **activity against SARS-CoV:** valinomycin, glycopeptide antibiotics, plant lectins, **hesperetin**, glycyrrhizin, aurintricarboxylic acid, chloroquine, niclosamide, nelfinavir and calpain inhibitors.

Inhibitory effects on SARS-CoV replication, with selectivity indexes of up to 100, and EC50 values as low as 1 µg/ml, **have been observed for a variety of compounds including** the vancomycin, eremomycin and teicoplanin aglycon derivatives [70], and the **mannose-specific plant lectins derived from *G. nivalis*, *Hippeastrum hybrid*[71]** and *Allium porrum* (leek) [72]. The mode of action of these compounds has not been assessed, but it is tempting to speculate that they interfere with the binding of the S glycoprotein to the host cells.

Isatis indigotica **root and phenolic Chinese herbs were frequently used for the prevention of SARS during the SARS outbreaks in China, Hong Kong and Taiwan.** *I. indigotica* root (*Radix isatidis*) is native to China. **From the** *I. indigotica* **root extracts several compounds, that is, indigo, sinigrin, aloe-emodin and hesperetin, were isolated that inhibited the cell-free and cell-based cleavage activity of the SARS Mpro (3CLpro)** at IC50 values ranging from 10 to 1000 µM [73]. The inhibitory effects on SARS-CoV replication in cell culture (i.e., Vero cells) were not determined in this study. The cytotoxicity was determined, however, and, based on the ratio of the CC50 to the IC50 (cell-based cleavage), **hesperetin appeared to be the most selective** (selectivity index: ~300) [73]."

De Clercq, Erik. "Potential antivirals and antiviral strategies against SARS coronavirus infections." *Expert review of anti-infective therapy* vol. 4,2 (2006): 291-302. doi:10.1586/14787210.4.2.291

"Antiviral activity of carbohydrate-binding agents against Nidovirales in cell culture"

"Coronaviruses are important human and animal pathogens, the relevance of which increased due **to the emergence of new human coronaviruses like SARS-CoV, HKU1 and NL63. Together with** toroviruses, arteriviruses, and roniviruses the coronaviruses belong to the order *Nidovirales*. **So far antivirals are hardly available to combat infections with viruses of this order.** Therefore, various antiviral strategies to counter nidoviral infections are under evaluation. Lectins, which bind to N-linked oligosaccharide elements of enveloped viruses, can be considered as a conceptionally new class of virus inhibitors. These agents were recently evaluated for their antiviral activity towards a variety of enveloped viruses and were shown in most cases to inhibit virus infection at low concentrations. However, limited knowledge is available for their efficacy towards nidoviruses. **In this article the application of the plant lectins *Hippeastrum* hybrid agglutinin (HHA), *Galanthus nivalis* agglutinin (GNA), *Cymbidium* sp. agglutinin (CA) and *Urtica dioica* agglutinin (UDA) as well as non-plant derived pradimicin-A (PRM-A) and cyanovirin-N (CV-N) as potential antiviral agents was evaluated.** Three antiviral tests were compared based on different evaluation principles: cell viability (MTT-based colorimetric assay), number of infected cells (immunoperoxidase assay) and amount of viral protein expression (luciferase-based assay). **The presence of carbohydrate-binding agents strongly inhibited coronaviruses (transmissible gastroenteritis virus, infectious bronchitis virus, feline coronaviruses serotypes I and II, mouse hepatitis virus), arteriviruses (equine arteritis virus and porcine respiratory and reproductive syndrome virus) and torovirus (equine Berne virus).** Remarkably, serotype II feline coronaviruses and arteriviruses were not inhibited by PRM-A, in contrast to the other viruses tested.

"We were able to show for UDA [*Urtica dioica* agglutinin] [stinging nettle rhizome] also a high antiviral efficacy against all evaluated *Nidovirales* except PRRSV."

van der Meer, F J U M et al. "Antiviral activity of carbohydrate-binding agents against Nidovirales in cell culture." *Antiviral research* vol. 76,1 (2007): 21-9. doi:10.1016/j.antiviral.2007.04.003

"An unusual lectin from stinging nettle (Urtica dioica) rhizomes"

"UDA induced considerable amounts of antiviral activity in the cell cultures. Moreover, the antiviral activity produced after stimulating lymphocytes with UDA was characterized by using specific antisera as being due solely to HuIFN-y (formerly called immune interferon)."

Peumans, Willy J. et al. "An unusual lectin from stinging nettle (Urtica dioica) rhizomes." *FEBS Letters* 177 (1984): n. pag.

"Effective inhibition of MERS-CoV infection by resveratrol"

"Resveratrol significantly inhibited MERS-CoV infection and prolonged cellular survival after virus infection. We also found that the expression of nucleocapsid (N) protein essential for MERS-CoV replication was decreased after resveratrol treatment. Furthermore, resveratrol

down-regulated the apoptosis induced by MERS-CoV in vitro. By consecutive administration of resveratrol, we were able to reduce the concentration of resveratrol while achieving inhibitory effectiveness against MERS-CoV."

"In this study, we first demonstrated that resveratrol is a potent anti-MERS agent in vitro. We perceive that resveratrol can be a potential antiviral agent against MERS-CoV infection in the near future."

Lin, Shih-Chao et al. "Effective inhibition of MERS-CoV infection by resveratrol." *BMC infectious diseases* vol. 17,1 144. 13 Feb. 2017, doi:10.1186/s12879-017-2253-8

"In vitro antiviral activity of fifteen plant extracts against avian infectious bronchitis virus"

"IB is a highly contagious respiratory and occasionally urogenital disease in chickens [1]. **IBV affects the upper respiratory tract** and reduces egg production [2]. **It is a coronavirus that belongs to the *Coronaviridae* family. IBV is an enveloped virus with a single-stranded positive-sense linear RNA molecule (approximately 27.6 kb in size) [3].**

IB has a wide geographical distribution and is diagnosed worldwide [1]. IB outbreaks continuously and results in economic losses in the poultry industry. **So far vaccination using inactivated or live vaccines [4] is regarded as the main method of prevention, but it is not having the desired effect [5,6,7]. The high level of mutations of IBV [8] leads to the emergence of new serotypes and genotypes, and limits the efficacy of routine prevention.**

Antiviral effect against IBV

According to the results of the antiviral effect assay, eight extracts were selected for determination of the virucidal effect. **The selected extracts of *S. montana, O. vulgare, M. piperita, M. officinalis, T. vulgaris, H. officinalis, S. officinalis* and *D. canadense* showed anti-IBV activity in two of the four methods. All eight extracts showed an antiviral effect prior to infection (method 1). Furthermore, seven of these showed antiviral activity during infection (method 2), while only the extract of *S. montana [Satureja montana]* [winter savory] showed anti-IBV activity after infection (method 4). *P. frutescens, N. cataria, E. purpurea, Ch. nobile* and *A. foeniculum* showed an antiviral effect only in the first method, while *G. macrorrhizum* and *A. archangelica* did not show an antiviral effect in any method (Table 1).**

The above-mentioned eight plant extracts demonstrating anti-IBV activity were selected for further investigation. The 50% effective concentration (EC50) was determined in cells grown for 4 days (prior to infection). The EC50 values of extracts of *S. montana, O. vulgare* [oregano], *M. piperita* [peppermint], *M. officinalis* [lemon balm], *T. vulgaris* [thyme], *H. officinalis, S. officinalis* and *D. canadense* were between 0.003 and 0.076 μg, however **S. officinalis [Salvia officinalis] appeared effective at the lowest concentration (0.003 μg)** (Table 2). SI of *M. piperita, O. vulgare,* and *T. vulgaris* extracts were 67.5, 65.0 and 63.1 respectively."

"Traditional Chinese Medicine in the Treatment of Patients Infected with 2019-New Coronavirus (SARS-CoV-2): A Review and Perspective"

"There are quite compelling evidences support the notion that TCM has beneficial effect in the treatment or prevention of SARS. For example, the rate of fatality in Hong Kong and Singapore was approximately 18%, while the rate for Beijing was initially more than 52% until the 5th of May and decreased gradually to 4%-1% after the 20th of May in 2003. The dramatic reduced fatality from late May in Beijing was believed to be associated with the use of TCM as a supplement to the conventional therapy [44]. Lau and colleagues reported that, during SARS outbreak, 1063 volunteers including 926 hospital workers and 37 laboratory technicians working in high-risk virus laboratories used a TCM herbal extract, namely *Sang Ju Yin* plus *Yu Ping Feng San*. Compared with the 0.4% of infection in the control group, none of TCM users infected. Furthermore, there was some evidence that *Sang Ju Yin* plus *Yu Ping Feng San* could modulate T cells in a manner to enhance host defense capacity [45, 46]. In a controlled clinical study, the supplementary treatment with TCM resulted in marked improvement of symptoms and shortened the disease course [47]. The clinical beneficial effect of TCM appears to be supported by laboratory studies."

TCM Compound (s)	Mode of action	Reference
Plant-derived phenolic compounds and Root extract of *Isatis indigotica*	Inhibit the cleavage activity of SARS-3CLpro enzyme	[57]
Water extract of *Houttuynia cordata*	Inhibit the viral SARS-3CLpro activity Block viral RNA-dependent RNA polymerase activity (RdRp) Immunomodulation	[54, 55]
Scutellarein and myricetin	Inhibit nsP13 by affecting the ATPase activity	[61]
Glycyrrhizin from *Glycyrrhizae radix*	Inhibit viral adsorption and penetration	[48, 75]
Herbacetin, quercetin, isobavaschalcone, 3-β-D-glucoside and helichrysetin	Inhibit cleavage activity of MERS-3CLpro enzyme	[60]
Tetrandrine, fangchinoline, and cepharanthine	Inhibit the expression of HCoV-OC43 spike and nucleocapsid protein. Immunomodulation	[106, 119]
Chinese Rhubarb extracts	Inhibit SARS-3CLpro activity	[53]
Flavonoids (For example: extracted from litchi seeds, herbacetin, rhoifolin, pectolinarin, quercetin, epigallocatechin gallate, and gallocatechin gallate)	Inhibit SARS-3CLpro activity	[56, 58, 59]
Quercetin and TSL-1 from *Toona sinensis* Roem	Inhibit the cellular entry of SARS-CoV	[76]
Emodin derived from genus *Rheum* and *Polygonum*	Inhibit interaction of SARS-CoV Spike protein and ACE2 Inhibit the 3a ion channel of coronavirus SARS-CoV and HCoV-OC43	[67, 72]
Kaempferol derivatives	Inhibit 3a ion channel of coronavirus	[73]
Baicalin from *Scutellaria baicalensis*	Inhibit Angiotensin-converting enzyme (ACE)	[44, 68]
Saikosaponins	Prevent the early stage of HCoV-22E9 infection, including viral attachment and penetration	[74]
Tetra-O-galloyl-β-D-glucose and luteolin, from *Galla chinensis* and *Veronica linariifolia* respectively	Avidly binds with surface spike protein of SARS-CoV	[71]

"The helicase protein is also considered as a potential target for the development of anti-HCoV (human coronavirus) agents. Yu *et al.* reported **scutellarein and myricetin potently inhibited the nsP13 (SARS-CoV helicase protein)** *in vitro* **by affecting the ATPase activity** [61]. The RNA- dependent RNA polymerase (RdRp), a key enzyme responsible for both positive and negative-strand RNA synthesis, also represents another potential druggable target. It was shown that the **extracts of** *Kang Du Bu Fei Tang* **(IC50:471.3 μg/mL),** *Sinomenium acutum* **(IC50:198.6 μg/mL),** *Coriolus versicolor* **[turkey tail mushroom] (IC50:108.4 μg/mL) and** *Ganoderma lucidum* **[reishi] (IC50:41.9 μg/mL) inhibited SARS-CoV RdRp in a dose- dependent manner** [54]. Wu *et al.* performed large- scale screening of existing drugs, natural products, and synthetic compounds (>10000 compounds) to identify effective anti-SARS-CoV agents through a cell-based assay with SARS virus and Vero E6 cells [62]. They found that ginsenoside-Rb1 isolated from *Panax ginseng*, aescin isolated from the horse chestnut tree, reserpine contained in the genus *Rauwolfia* and extracts of *eucalyptus* and *Lonicera japonica* inhibited SARS-CoV replication at non-toxic concentrations [62].

Same as SARS-CoV and HCoV-NL63, SARS-CoV-2 uses host receptor ACE2 for the cellular entrance [63-66]. Therefore, TCM with the capacity to target ACE2 holds the promise to prevent the infection of SARS-CoV-2. Emodin from genus *Rheum* and *Polygonum* [67], baicalin from in *Scutellaria baicalensis* [44, 68], **nicotianamine from foodstuff (especially "soybean ACE2 inhibitor (ACE2iSB)")** [69], scutellarin [70], tetra-*O*-galloyl-β-D-glucose (TGG) from *Galla chinensis* and luteolin from *Veronicalina riifolia* [71] markedly inhibited the interaction of SARS-CoV S-protein and ACE2. However, the anti-SARS-CoV activity of these compounds remain to be evaluated. In addition, inhibition of the 3a ion channel by emodin [72] or kaempferol derivatives-juglanin [73] could potentially prevent the viral release from the infected cells. **Saikosaponins** [74], **glycyrrhizin** [48, 75], **quercetin and TSL-1 extracted from** *Toona sinensis* **Roem** [76] **purportedly had potent anti-SARS-CoV effects by inhibition of viral cellular entry, adsorption, and penetration.**

Overwhelming inflammatory responses are attributable to the deaths of patients with infection of SARS-CoV, or MERS-CoV, or COVID-19. Thus, anti-inflammatory agents presumably could reduce the severity and mortality rate [77]. *Shuang Huang Lian,* **a TCM herbal product prepared from** *Lonicerae japonicae* **Flos,** *Scutellariae radix* **and** *Fructus Forsythiae,* **purportedly had the activity to inhibit SARS-CoV-2** [78]. **Interestingly, We have shown that this herbal preparation potently inhibited staphylococcal toxic shock syndrome toxin 1 (TSST-1)-induced production of cytokines (IL-1β, IL-6, TNF-α, IFN-γ) and chemokines (MIP-1α, MIP-1β and MCP-1) by peripheral blood mononuclear cell (PBMC)** [79]. **In line with our results, this herbal product was shown to markedly reduced the transcriptional and translational levels of inflammatory cytokines TNF-α, IL-1β, and IL-6 in lipopolysaccharide-stimulated murine alveolar macrophages** [80]. Indirubin is an active ingredient of a TCM preparation *Dang Gui Long Hui Pill,* had strong antiviral and immunomodulatory effects, as shown by a study based on the observation of influenza H5N1 virus-infected human macrophages and type-I alveolar epithelial cells [81]. *Lian Hua Qing Wen Capsule* **was reported to have** *in vitro* **activity in inhibition of propagation of various influenza viruses. This TCM herbal product not only blocked the early stages of influenza virus infection but also inhibited virus-induced gene expression of IL-6, IL-8, TNF-a, IP-10, and MCP-1** [82]. **Additionally, a study by Dong *et al.* reported that the levels of IL-8, TNF-α, IL-17, and IL-23 in the sputum and of IL-8 and IL-17 in the blood were markedly decreased after *Lian Hua Qing Wen Capsule* treatment in patients with acute exacerbation of chronic obstructive pulmonary disease** [83]. A self-control study by Poon *et al.* showed that the administration of the TCM herbal formulas (*Sang Ju Yin* and *Yu Ping Feng San*) may have beneficial immunomodulatory effects for the prevention of viral infections including SARS-CoV [46].

Moreover, a number of anti-coronaviral agents have been identified from TCM herbs, although the mechanisms of action have not yet been elucidated. For example, extracts from *Lycoris radiata*, *Artemisia annua*, *Pyrrosia lingua*, and *Lindera aggregate* possessed the anti-SARS-CoV activity [84], **3β-Friedelanol isolated from *Euphorbia neriifolia* [85], Blancoxanthone isolated from the roots of *Calophyllum blancoi* [86] exhibited anti-HCoV-229E activity.**"

Yang, Yang et al. "Traditional Chinese Medicine in the Treatment of Patients Infected with 2019-New Coronavirus (SARS-CoV-2): A Review and Perspective." *International journal of biological sciences* vol. 16,10 1708-1717. 15 Mar. 2020, doi:10.7150/ijbs.45538

"Echinacea—A Source of Potent Antivirals for Respiratory Virus Infections"

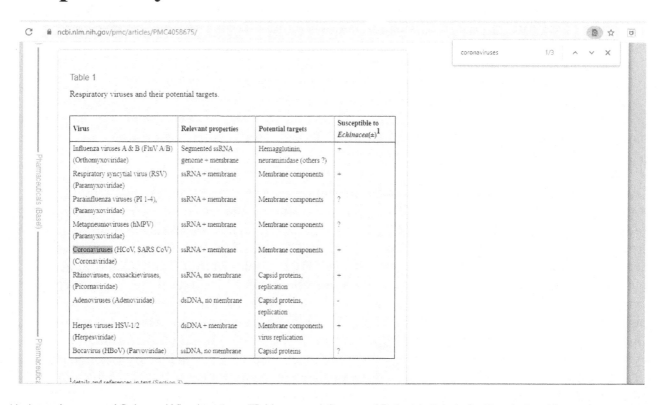

Table 1

Respiratory viruses and their potential targets.

Virus	Relevant properties	Potential targets	Susceptible to Echinacea(±)[1]
Influenza viruses A & B (FluV A/B) (Orthomyxoviridae)	Segmented ssRNA genome + membrane	Hemagglutinin, neuraminidase (others ?)	+
Respiratory syncytial virus (RSV) (Paramyxoviridae)	ssRNA + membrane	Membrane components	+
Parainfluenza viruses (PI 1-4), (Paramyxoviridae)	ssRNA + membrane	Membrane components	?
Metapneumoviruses (hMPV) (Paramyxoviridae)	ssRNA + membrane	Membrane components	?
Coronaviruses (HCoV, SARS CoV) (Coronaviridae)	ssRNA + membrane	Membrane components	+
Rhinoviruses, coxsackieviruses, (Picornaviridae)	ssRNA, no membrane	Capsid proteins, replication	+
Adenoviruses (Adenoviridae)	dsDNA, no membrane	Capsid proteins, replication	-
Herpes viruses HSV-1/2 (Herpesviridae)	dsDNA + membrane	Membrane components virus replication	+
Bocavirus (HBoV) (Parvoviridae)	ssDNA, no membrane	Capsid proteins	?

[1]details and references in text (Section 3)

Hudson, James, and Selvarani Vimalanathan. "Echinacea—A Source of Potent Antivirals for Respiratory Virus Infections." *Pharmaceuticals* vol. 4,7 1019–1031. 13 Jul. 2011, doi:10.3390/ph4071019

"High-Throughput Screening and Identification

of Potent Broad-Spectrum Inhibitors of Coronaviruses"

"Furthermore, we identified seven compounds (**lycorine**, emetine, monensin sodium, mycophenolate mofetil, mycophenolic acid, phenazopyridine, and pyrvinium pamoate) as **broad-spectrum inhibitors according to their strong inhibition of replication by four CoVs *in vitro* at low-micromolar concentrations.** Additionally, we found that emetine blocked MERS-CoV entry according to pseudovirus entry assays and that lycorine protected BALB/c mice against HCoV-OC43-induced lethality by decreasing viral load in the central nervous system. **This represents the first demonstration of *in vivo* real-time bioluminescence imaging to monitor the effect of lycorine on the spread and distribution of HCoV-OC43 in a mouse model. These results offer critical information supporting the development of an effective therapeutic strategy against CoV infection.**"

Shen, Liang et al. "High-Throughput Screening and Identification of Potent Broad-Spectrum Inhibitors of Coronaviruses." *Journal of virology* vol. 93,12 e00023-19. 29 May. 2019, doi:10.1128/JVI.00023-19

"Eupatorium fortunei and Its Components Increase Antiviral Immune Responses against RNA Viruses"

"Also, according to recent research results, **quercetin has been shown to protect against** the entry of influenza A virus (Wu et al., 2015) and interaction between human respiratory syncytial virus M2-1 protein (Teixeira et al., 2017), have anti-HSV-1 and anti-HSV-2 properties (Lee et al., 2017), **and inhibit coronavirus** and dengue virus infection (Chiow et al., 2016)."

Choi, Jang-Gi et al. "*Eupatorium fortunei* and Its Components Increase Antiviral Immune Responses against RNA Viruses." *Frontiers in pharmacology* vol. 8 511. 3 Aug. 2017, doi:10.3389/fphar.2017.00511

COVID-19 Epidemiology, Clinical Features, Hypothetical Regimens

by Collin Gow, C.N.C. (3/26/2020)

OVERVIEW

COVID-19 Fatality Rate by AGE:

*__Death Rate__ = (number of deaths / number of cases) = **probability of dying if infected by the virus** (%). This probability differs depending on the age group. The percentages shown below do not have to add up to 100%, as they **do NOT represent share of deaths by age group**. Rather, it represents, for a person in a given age group, the **risk of dying** if infected with COVID-19.

AGE	DEATH RATE confirmed cases	DEATH RATE all cases
80+ years old	21.9%	14.8%
70-79 years old		8.0%
60-69 years old		3.6%
50-59 years old		1.3%
40-49 years old		0.4%
30-39 years old		0.2%
20-29 years old		0.2%
10-19 years old		0.2%
0-9 years old		no fatalities

*__Death Rate__ = (number of deaths / number of cases) = **probability of dying if infected by the virus** (%).

Sources:
The Epidemiological Characteristics of an Outbreak of 2019 Novel Coronavirus Diseases (COVID-19) - China CCDC, February 17 2020

Report of the WHO-China Joint Mission on Coronavirus Disease 2019 (COVID-19) [Pdf] - World Health Organization, Feb. 28, 2020

Annual Risk Of Death During One's Lifetime

DISEASE AND ACCIDENTAL CAUSES OF DEATHS	ANNUAL DEATHS	DEATH RISK DURING ONE'S LIFETIME
Heart disease	652,486	1 in 5
Cancer	553,888	1 in 7
Stroke	150,074	1 in 24
Hospital Infections	99,000	1 in 38
Flu	59,664	1 in 63
Car accidents	44,757	1 in 84
Suicide	31,484	1 in 119
Accidental poisoning	19,456	1 in 193
MRSA (resistant bacteria)	19,000	1 in 197
Falls	17,229	1 in 218
Drowning	3,306	1 in 1,134
Bike accident	762	1 in 4,919
Air/space accident	742	1 in 5,051

Sources: All accidental death information from National Safety Council. Disease death information from Centers for Disease Control and Prevention. Shark fatality data provided by the International Shark Attack File.

Lifetime risk is calculated by dividing 2003 population (290,850,005) by the number of deaths, divided by 77.6, the life expectancy of a person born in 2003.

There's a .2% chance of dying from COVID-19 if you get it and if age 30-39. That's a 1 in 500 chance of dying from it if you get it. But that's probably the chance if you are under the care of a physician in an allopathic care setting, not if you're on natural meds. And the chance that you will get it is not 100% so it lowers the overall chance of dying from it to even less than .2%. But, let's just use the 1 in 500 number to give the benefit of the doubt that we are all going to get it and that we are all going to be treated allopathically. **A 1 in 500 chance of dying from corona is less of a chance than dying from falling, MRSA, accidental poisoning, suicide, car accidents, flu, hospital infections, stroke, cancer, and heart disease! If driving your car is more hazardous than corona, then why the big hubub about it?**

Symptoms: fever (most common symptom), cough, myalgia (muslce pain), fatigue, sore throat, mucus production, headache, trouble breathing, haemoptysis (coughing up blood), diarrhea.[1,2] **If symptoms become unbearable, seek immediate medical attention!**

Complications: pneumonia, lymphopenia (low lymphocyte count), leucopenia (low white blood cell count), cardiac injury, kidney injury, shock, secondary infection, respiratory distress, RNAaemia, prolonged prothrombin time (blood taking too long to clot), elevated D-Dimer (byproducts of fibrinolysis), hypoxia (low O_2).[1,2]

Other Clinical Features: high plasma concentrations of IL1B, IL1RA, IL7, IL8, IL9, IL10, basic FGF, GCSF, GMCSF, IFNγ, IP10, MCP1, MIP1A, MIP1B, PDGF, TNFα, and VEG upon admission.[1,2]

Conventional Treatment: antivirals (oseltamivir, etc.), antibiotics, corticosteroids, ventialtion, nasal cannula, kidney transplant.[1,2]

Contraindications: ACE inhibitors & angiotensin receptor blocker meds may ↑ infect risk (Diaz et al.)

MUST HAVES

1. Boost the immune system – **Pick 2 of the following and double the doses recommended on the bottles or do the max dose the bottle suggests:** echinacea, astragalus, mushrooms, cat's claw, zinc (hydroxychloroquine works by pushing zinc into the cells), vitamin A, C, D3, E, selenium, colostrum, hGh, multivitamin. **Or pick 1 of the following and double the dose recommended on the bottle (but don't double the dose on the Source Naturals Wellness Formula):** Bluebonnet Wellness Support, Solaray Under the Weather Plus, Source Naturals Wellness Formula, Megafood Acute Defense, or Gaia Quick Defense. These formulas have many immune boosting ingredients in one product.

2. Take antivirals studied against coronaviruses and/or HIV (HIV-1-like inserts have been found in COVID-19)[3] – **Pick 1 of the following and quadruple the dose recommended on the bottle or pick 2 options and only double the dose on each bottle. Studied against coronaviruses:** red algae,[4] *Artemisia annua* (wormwood),[5] thyme, oregano, and peppermint,[6] licorice,[7] nettle root,[8] horse chestnut,[9] or quercetin.[10] **Studied against HIV:** silver,[11] spirulina,[12] olive leaf,[13] *Artemisia annua*,[14] andrographis,[15] elderberry,[16] reishi.[17] **Other antivirals:** shilajit, goldenseal, agarikon, lysine. **I do not recommend high doses of garlic, only minimal to average doses** as it thins the blood too much for this particular issue.

3. Reduce inflammation in the lungs (Dr.s use corticosteroids as part of their treatment of COVID-19) – **Pick 1 of the following and double, triple, or quadruple the dose recommended on the bottle:** boswellia, black seed oil, ginger, turmeric, rosemary, bromelain, pancreatin, green tea, tart cherry, white willow, omega 3s, etc. **Or pick 1 of the following and double the dose recommended on the bottle:** New Chapter Zyflamend, Crystal Star Inflama Relief, Life Seasons Inflamma – X, Michael's Recovery Zymes or Wobenzym.

4. Take a respiratory product – **Pick 1 of the following and use as directed, double, triple, or quadruple the dose recommended on the bottle:** oregano oil, black seed oil, peppermint, eucalyptus, NAC, Terry Naturally Bronchial Clear Liquid, Dr. Chi Bamboo Extract, Old Indian Wild Cherry Bark syrup, Natural Factors Lung Bronchial and Sinus, Vitality Works Respir-Ease, (or herbs such as elecampane, lobelia, yerba santa, wild cherry bark, horehound, hyssop, mullein, marshmallow, thyme, etc. **And/or nebulize glutathione (theranaturals brand) or silver or use a salt inhaler.**

5. Boost oxygen levels without taking excessive iron (iron may feed pathogens) (hypoxia is a complication of COVID-19 infection, hence ventilator and nasal cannula use in patients) – **Pick 1 of the following and double or triple the dose recommended on the bottle:** Chlorophyll, Chlorella, Chi Oxypower, Cordyceps, Rhodiola, Sun Warrior Liquid Light, Restore, CoQ10.

OPTIONAL

6. Take a febrifuge or antipyretic (fever reducer) (only if temperature goes above 104 degrees) - **Pick 1 of the following and double the dose recommended on the bottle:** ginger, peppermint, feverfew, cayenne, wormwood, black pepper, andrographis, yarrow, catnip, bergamot, white willow, Indian barberry, garlic, sage, holy basil, bitter melon, blood root, boneset, buchu, fenugreek, hops, horse chestnut, basically any spicy or bitter herb.

7. Boost vitamin K1 and calcium levels to assist with blood clotting (PTT and D-Dimer are elevated in COVID-19 patients) – **Follow the directions on the bottle:** drink a greens powder or eat lots of vegetables or take a minimum of 90mcg (female) or 120mcg (male) vitamin K1 per day either in or with a calcium supplement. New Chapter Bone Strength or Country Life Bone Solid are good choices. **These do not thicken the blood indiscriminately, they are only activated when there is an injury to the blood vessels.**

8. Strengthen capillaries (bleeding into the lungs may occur with acute COVID-19 infection) – **Follow the directions on the bottle or in some cases take less than recommended:** horse chestnut, butchers broom, pine bark extract/pycnogenol, silica or Dr. Chi Bamboo Extract, collagen, Solaray Circulegs or Nature's Way Vein Support. **I do not recommend high doses of grapeseed extract in this instance, normal/average doses are ok.** Horse Chestnut best choice at it is also studied to be antiviral against coronaviruses.[9]

9. Keep the liver, lymphatic system, and kidneys clean (organ overload/failure may occur in COVID-19 infection) – **Pick 1 of the following and follow the suggested use on the bottle or take less:** burdock, yellow dock, dandelion, red clover, milk thistle, artichoke, red root, echinacea, chlorophyll, cornsilk, cleavers, buchu, parsley, juniper, NAC, glutathione, broccoli seed extract. **Or Pick 1 of the following formulas and use as suggested on the bottle or take less:** Lymphatonic by Herbs Etc, NOW Liver Renew, Gaia Liver Cleanse, Solaray Skin (a lymphatic/blood cleanser), Solaray Tetra Cleanse, Solaray Kidney.

Other Tips: Drink extra water to keep fever down, check temperature regularly, **wash hands, wear an N95 mask** if you must go outside, **self-quarantine. Do not go into a health food store.** Call them and **have a friend or family member that hasn't been around you pick up your order.**

Hypothetical Regimen 1:
1. **Source Naturals Wellness Formula (capsules)** – 2 caps, 3X/DAY with food
2. **Vibrant Health Gigartina** – 4 caps, 2X/DAY with food
3. **Terry Naturally Bosmed** – 2 softgels, 3X/DAY with food
4. **Old Indian Wild Cherry Bark Syrup** – 2 Tbsp, 2X/DAY
5. **World Organic Liquid Chlorophyll** – 1 Tbsp, 2X/DAY
6. **2 tea bags peppermint,** 2X/DAY only if temp. above 104 degrees
7. **New Chapter Bone Strength** – 1 slim tab, 3X/DAY with food
8. **Nature's Way Vein Support** – 1 capsule/DAY
9. **Liver/Lymphatic/Kidney cleanse may not be needed**

Hypothetical Regimen 2:
1. **Gaia Echinacea Supreme (Do not need to double the dose on this one as the bottle already recommends high doses)** – 4 caps, 4X/DAY (highest dose recommended on the bottle)
   NOW OptiZinc – 1 cap, 2X/DAY with food
2. **Natural Factors Oregano Oil softgels** – 1 softgel, 4X/DAY with food

3. **Crystal Star Inflama Relief** – 2 caps, 4X/DAY with food
4. **Country Life NAC 750mg** – 2 caps, 2X/DAY on empty stomach
5. **Chi Oxypower** – 3 caps, 2X/DAY with food
6. **Febrifuge/Antipyretic may not be needed**
7. **Solgar vitamin K1 100mcg** – 1 tab/DAY
8. **Country Life Pycnogenol 50mg** – 1/DAY with food
9. **Liver/Lymphatic/Kidney cleanse may not be needed**

Hypothetical Regimen 3:
1. **Megafood Women's One Daily Multi** – 1 tab, 2X/DAY
   Immune Tree Colostrum Powder – 1 tsp, 2X/DAY
2. **Sovereign Silver** – 1 tsp, 7X/DAY
3. **Solaray Ginger** – 2 caps, 3X/DAY with food
4. **Terry Naturally Bronchial Clear Liquid** – 2 tsp, 2X/DAY
5. **Health Force Chlorella** – 1 tsp, 2X/DAY
6. **Febrifuge/Antipyretic may not be needed**
7. **K1/Calcium may not be needed**
8. **Dr. Chi Bamboo Extract** – 2 caps, 3X/DAY with food
9. **Liver/Lymphatic/Kidney cleanse may not be needed**

Hypothetical Regimen 4:
1. **Bluebonnet Wellness Support** – 2 tabs, 2X/DAY with food
2. **Solaray Horse Chestnut Extract** – 1 cap, 2X/DAY
   Oregon's Wild Harvest Licorice – 3 caps, 2X/DAY
3. **Michael's Recovery Zymes** – 3 tabs, 2X/DAY on empty stomach
4. **Heritage Store Black Seed Oil** – 1 tsp, 2X/DAY with food
5. **Sun Warrior Liquid Light** – 1 capful, 2X/DAY with food
6. **Febrifuge/Antipyretic may not be needed**
7. **Bluebonnet Organic Greens Powder** – 1 scoop/DAY
8. **Capillary product may not be needed**
9. **Liver/Lymphatic/Kidney cleanse may not be needed**

Hypothetical Regimen 5:
1. **Host Defense Stamets 7 Powder** – 1 tsp, 2X/DAY with food
   Trace Mineral Research Power Pack Vitamin C packets – 1, 2X/DAY with food
2. **Gaia Olive Leaf Capsules** – 2 caps, 2X/DAY with food
   Gaia Elderberry Syrup – 2 tsp, 2X/DAY
3. **Terry Naturally Curamed 750** – 1 softgel, 3X/DAY with food
4. **Vitality Works Respir-Ease -** 1 dropperful, 3X/DAY
5. **Gaia Rhodiola Capsules** – 2 caps, 2X/DAY
6. **2 tea bags ginger**, 2X/DAY only if temp. above 104 degrees
7. **Country Life vitamin K1 100mcg** – 1 tab/DAY
8. **Harmonic Innerprizes Silica** – 1 capsule/DAY with food
9. **Herbs Etc Lymphatonic** – 1 dropperful/DAY
   Or World Organic Liquid Chlorophyll – 1 Tbsp/DAY

Hypothetical Regimen 6:
1. **Gaia Quick Defense** – 4 caps, 2X/DAY
2. **Sunfood Shilajit Powder** – 1/8th tsp, 2X/DAY with food

3. **New Chapter Zyflamend** – 2 caps, 2X/DAY with food
4. **Natural Factors Lung Bronchial and Sinus** – 2 tabs, 3X/DAY
5. **Host Defense Cordyceps Capsules** – 2 caps, 2X/DAY
6. **Febrifuge/Antipyretic may not be needed**
7. **Spirulina Powder** – 1 tsp/DAY
8. **Sun Warrior Collagen or Garden of Life Beauty Collagen** – 1 scoop/DAY
9. **Liver/Lymphatic/Kidney cleanse may not be needed**

Foods: Limit processed foods and refined sugars. Limit high arginine foods (chocolate and nuts). Limit iron intake from supplements. Limit dairy, meat, and other animal foods (organ meats are ok). Eat mushrooms, garlic, onions, ginger, peppers, fermented foods, manuka honey, citrus fruits, seaweed (especially dulse), brazil nuts, cooked oysters, pumpkin seeds, nutritional yeast, and puer or black tea.[18]

References:

1. Huang, Chaolin & Wang, Yeming & Li, Xingwang & Ren, Lili & Zhao, Jianping & Hu, Yi & Zhang, Li & Fan, Guohui & Xu, Jiuyang & Gu, Xiaoying & Cheng, Zhenshun & Yu, Ting & Xia, Jiaan & Wei, Yuan & Wu, Wenjuan & Xie, Xuelei & Yin, Wen & Li, Hui & Liu, Min & Cao, Bin. (2020). Clinical features of patients infected with 2019 novel coronavirus in Wuhan, China. The Lancet. 395. 10.1016/S0140-6736(20)30183-5.
2. Cao, Min & Zhang, Dandan & Wang, Youhua & Lu, Yunfei & Zhu, Xiangdong & Li, Ying & Xue, Honghao & Lin, Yunxiao & Zhang, Min & Sun, Yiguo & Yang, Zongguo & Shi, Jia & Wang, Yi & Zhou, Chang & Dong, Yidan & Liu, Ping & Dudek, Steven & Xiao, Zhen & Lu, Hongzhou & Peng, Longping. (2020). Clinical Features of Patients Infected with the 2019 Novel Coronavirus (COVID-19) in Shanghai, China. 10.1101/2020.03.04.20030395.
3. Pradhan, Prashant & Pandey, Ashutosh & Mishra, Akhilesh & Gupta, Parul & Tripathi, Praveen & Menon, Manoj & Gomes, James & Perumal, Vivekanandan & Kundu, Bishwajit. (2020). Uncanny similarity of unique inserts in the 2019-nCoV spike protein to HIV-1 gp120 and Gag. 10.1101/2020.01.30.927871.
4. Lee, C. Griffithsin, a Highly Potent Broad-Spectrum Antiviral Lectin from Red Algae: From Discovery to Clinical Application. *Mar. Drugs* 2019, *17*, 567.
5. Lin LT, Hsu WC, Lin CC. Antiviral natural products and herbal medicines. *J Tradit Complement Med.* 2014;4(1):24–35. doi:10.4103/2225-4110.124335
6. Lelešius, Raimundas & Karpovaitė, Agneta & Mickienė, Rūta & Drevinskas, Tomas & Tiso, Nicola & Ragazinskiene, Ona & Kubilienė, Loreta & Maruska, Audrius & Salomskas, Algirdas. (2019). In vitro antiviral activity of fifteen plant extracts against avian infectious bronchitis virus. BMC Veterinary Research. 15. 10.1186/s12917-019-1925-6.
7. Cinatl, Jindrich & Morgenstern, B & Bauer, G & Chandra, Prof & Rabenau, Holger & Doerr, Hans Wilhelm. (2003). Glycyrrhizin, an active component of liquorice roots, and replication of SARS-associated coronavirus. Lancet. 361. 2045-6. 10.1016/S0140-6736(03)13615-X.
8. van der Meer, Frank & de Haan, Cornelis & Schuurman, N & Haijema, Bert & Peumans, W & Damme, Els & Delputte, Peter & Balzarini, J & Egberink, H.F.. (2007). Antiviral activity of carbohydrate-binding agents against Nidovirales in cell culture. Antiviral research. 76. 21-9. 10.1016/j.antiviral.2007.04.003.
9. Yang Y, Islam MS, Wang J, Li Y, Chen X. Traditional Chinese Medicine in the Treatment of Patients Infected with 2019-New Coronavirus (SARS-CoV-2): A Review and Perspective. *Int J Biol Sci* 2020; 16(10):1708-1717. doi:10.7150/ijbs.45538. Available

from http://www.ijbs.com/v16p1708.htm

10. Choi, Jang-Gi & Lee, Heeeun & Hwang, Youn-Hwan & Lee, Jong-Soo & Cho, Won-Kyung & Ma, Jin. (2017). Eupatorium fortunei and Its Components Increase Antiviral Immune Responses against RNA Viruses. Frontiers in Pharmacology. 8. 511. 10.3389/fphar.2017.00511.

11. Lara HH, Ayala-Nuñez NV, Ixtepan-Turrent L, Rodriguez-Padilla C. Mode of antiviral action of silver nanoparticles against HIV-1. *J Nanobiotechnology*. 2010;8:1. Published 2010 Jan 20. doi:10.1186/1477-3155-8-1

12. S. Ayehunie, A. Belay, T. W. Baba, and R. M. Ruprecht, "Inhibition of HIV-1 replication by an aqueous extract of *Spirulina platensis (Arthrospira platensis),*" *Journal of Acquired Immune Deficiency Syndromes and Human Retrovirology*, vol. 18, no. 1, pp. 7–12, 1998.

13. Lee-Huang S, Huang PL, Zhang D, et al. Discovery of small-molecule HIV-1 fusion and integrase inhibitors oleuropein and hydroxytyrosol: Part I. fusion [corrected] inhibition [published correction appears in Biochem Biophys Res Commun. 2007 May 18;356(4):1068]. *Biochem Biophys Res Commun*. 2007;354(4):872–878. doi:10.1016/j.bbrc.2007.01.071

14. Salehi B, Kumar NVA, Şener B, et al. Medicinal Plants Used in the Treatment of Human Immunodeficiency Virus. *Int J Mol Sci*. 2018;19(5):1459. Published 2018 May 14. doi:10.3390/ijms19051459

15. Jayakumar T, Hsieh CY, Lee JJ, Sheu JR. Experimental and Clinical Pharmacology of Andrographis paniculata and Its Major Bioactive Phytoconstituent Andrographolide. *Evid Based Complement Alternat Med*. 2013;2013:846740. doi:10.1155/2013/846740

16. Fink, R. C., Roschek, B., & Alberte, R. S. (2009). HIV Type-1 Entry Inhibitors with a New Mode of Action. Antiviral Chemistry and Chemotherapy, 243–255. https://doi.org/10.1177/095632020901900604

17. Lindequist U, Niedermeyer TH, Jülich WD. The pharmacological potential of mushrooms. *Evid Based Complement Alternat Med*. 2005;2(3):285–299. doi:10.1093/ecam/neh107

18. Chen CN, Lin CP, Huang KK, et al. Inhibition of SARS-CoV 3C-like Protease Activity by Theaflavin-3,3'-digallate (TF3). *Evid Based Complement Alternat Med*. 2005;2(2):209–215. doi:10.1093/ecam/neh081

Amazing Immunity Supplements and Foods Available at Health Food Stores!

(Availability may vary)

Collin Gow, C.N.C.

4/4/20

Immunity Supplements

1. **Anti-V** (Natural Factors)
2. **Oregano oil** (Natural Factors)
3. **Echinacea**
4. **Quick Defense** (Gaia)
5. **Mushroom Caps and Powders** (Host Defense, Health Force, Solaray)
6. **Olive Leaf** (Gaia)
7. **Silver Hydrosol** (Sovereign Silver)
8. **ACF, ACF Extra Strength, ACF Children's** (Buried Treasure)
9. **Bronchial Soothe** (Nature's Way)
10. **Gigartina or Red Algae**
11. **Greens Powders**
12. **Shilajit Powder** (Sunfood)
13. **Colostrum** (Immune Tree)
14. **Immune Extra** (Allera Health Products)
15. **Moducare** (Wakunaga)
16. **Immune Health Basics** (Portals Pharma Inc.)
17. **Vitamin C**
18. **GSE** (Nutribiotic)
19. **Probiotics** (Megafood, Probulin, Vital Flora, Dr. Ohhira's)
20. **Oxypower, Bamboo, Reishi** (Dr. Chi)

Immunity Foods

1. **Mushrooms** (do not buy portobello) (fresh bulk and Mother Earth brand are good)
2. **Raw Garlic and Raw Onions**
3. **Ginger, Peppermint, or Licorice tea**
4. **Hot Peppers**
5. **Yams, Sweet potatoes, Squashes**
6. **Fermented foods** (water kefir, coconut water kefir, goat milk kefir, kombucha, umeboshi plums, tempeh, miso, goat or sheep milk yogurt, vegan yogurts, sauerkraut, kimchi, apple cider vinegar)
7. **Manuka Honey or Regular Raw Honey**
8. **Citrus fruits**
9. **Seaweed** (especially Maine Coast dulse)
10. **Brazil nuts** (bulk) **and Pumpkin Seeds** (Bulk)
11. **Canned Oysters** (Crown Prince)
12. **Liver or Liver Powder**

13. **Nutritional Yeast** (Bob's Redmill)
14. **Puer or Black Tea**
15. **Bulk Herbs and Spices** (Turmeric, Nettle, Peppermint, Oregano, Ginger)
16. **Fresh Herbs** (Thyme, Sage, Rosemary, Basil, Dill)
17. **Coconut Butter, Shredded Coconut, Coconut Oil**
18. **Celtic or Himalayan Salt**
19. **Oats**
20. **Fresh Juices and Smoothies**

Do Respirators, Surgical Masks, Or Face Coverings Protect Against COVID-19?: Taking the Science and Question in Context

Collin Gow, C.N.C.

June 18, 2020

This article presents information on the pros and cons of wearing face masks and asks the question whether or not they should be part of a healthy approach by the **public** to protecting themselves from COVID-19. **While some of the studies presented within this article talk about masks in medical settings, this article does not address the subject of mask-wearing in medical settings by medical professionals to a large degree, rather it focuses on mask wearing by the public**. I must also preface this article by saying that whether or not one wears a mask is a personal choice. Each person's situation is different and each person should decide for themselves whether or not wearing a mask is the right choice for them and their beliefs about the world. If one chooses to wear or not wear a mask to protect themselves, that's their prerogative. If one chooses to wear or not wear a mask to protect others that's their prerogative. If one chooses to wear or not wear a mask to protect themselves and others that's their prerogative. If one chooses to wear or not wear a mask for social comfort or for other reasons that's their prerogative. **You are responsible for your own health and your own decisions**. I am not liable for what you choose to do. I only present information for your consideration. **You should always talk to your doctor/naturopath before making any changes.** It's also important to know that the science and opinions and policies on a given subject constantly change based on new, developing information. Despite the wishful thinking of some folks, **the science is NEVER settled**. There is no such thing as settled and this article is not to be construed as a final say on the topic of mask-wearing. Moving on.

The **CDC** currently recommends that "**everyone**" over the **age of 2** wear a cloth **face covering** in public unless they have trouble breathing or are unconscious or cannot remove the mask without assistance. This updated recommendation overturns their previous recommendation that only those who are sick or taking care of the sick should wear one. It is not recommended by the CDC to wear a **respirator** or **surgical mask** as those are to be reserved for healthcare workers and first responders. The **WHO** originally advised the public not to wear masks, like the CDC, unless they are sick or caring for the sick, for fear they would use up supplies needed by medical workers and create a "false sense of security" and now they are saying that the general public should wear a mask in public places where physical distancing is difficult to maintain and in settings of high population density. This updated recommendation comes with a caveat that they admit: "At the present time, the widespread use of masks by healthy people in the community setting is not yet supported by high quality or direct scientific evidence and there are potential benefits and harms to consider", (WHO, 2020). **The U.S. surgeon general**, a member of **The Whitehouse Coronavirus Task Force**, originally cautioned against masks for those who are not ill or taking care of the ill but has now urged the public to wear face coverings, lockstep in line with the CDC. A variety of pundits appearing on **mainstream media television** have recommended that the public wear face masks. Many **governors** have been following CDC recommendations and urging the use of masks too. **Our fellow face mask wearing Americans** are shaming others who are not wearing them, making them feel like they're selfish murders for not wearing one. With such a disproportionate cry of passionate voices on one side of the subject, often, but not always, blindly following and championing the dictums of our leaders and the rhetoric of the mainstream, the establishment, and the status quo, perhaps it is time to level the playing field, show some actual **scientific research** on the topic, show both sides of the divide, and think about the prospect of mask-wearing in a **broader context**, rather than just unquestioningly accepting the chants and bleats of the herd. Gandhi said, "even if you are a minority of one, the truth is the truth". So lets question. Let's find out the truth. (I am not saying that everyone who wears a mask is blindly accepting what they've been told and doing no research for themselves, nor am I shaming people who are wearing masks. I'm only saying that *some* people are blindly accepting and I am only advocating the questioning of the status quo.)

Let's start with the broader context first, then move on to the scientific research on respirators and masks. If the majority of the public and the majority of the people in positions of power in America are either going along with or at least heeding the CDC and WHO's advice, then perhaps we should investigate these agencies a little bit to see if what they are saying is sound and sage advice or not. **Should we trust the CDC or the WHO or the Coronavirus Task Force or the mass media or governors?** The CDC is a U.S. government agency, but let's remember, in America, there is probably no such thing as government, only the illusion of government, as billionaires and corporations likely own our government through their obscene and exorbitant "donations" and lobbying powers. For example, **Bill Gates gave the CDC $1 million in 2003, $30 million in 2013/14 and he is now the 2nd largest contributor of funding to the WHO behind the U.S. government after giving a combined $20 million to groups that included them and the CDC in 2020 to combat COVID-19. He has given the WHO at least $327 million to date. Don't you think that has an effect on the CDC's suggestions?** The WHO is a United Nations agency. The U.N. has an agenda on record called **Agenda 21 aka Agenda 2030** which seeks to control and reduce the population, vaccinate everyone, sterilize people, take away private land, eliminate rights and freedoms, and establish a global government, under the guise of creating a sustainable future for the planet. If you believe that vaccines are healthy and good for you and are capable of saving the world, well, then you just haven't done enough of your own research, haven't studied the history of vaccination, don't know that **sanitation cured polio, not the vaccine**, don't understand the regulations on vaccines or what they actually mean when they say that they are "safe and effective", don't realize that you cannot legally sue a vaccine company for damages to your child from a vaccine, aren't aware that **getting the flu vaccine may increase your risk of getting coronaviruses by 36%,**[1] or maybe you think that **cancer causing viruses such as SV40, cancer causing chemicals such as formaldehyde (given the highest possible hazard rating there is on the EWG website), demyelinating, nervous system destroying metals like mercury and aluminum, fetal diploid cells, monkey kidney cells, bovine calf serum, chicken embryos, coronaviruses from dogs**, and the rest of the slew of toxic compounds they contain are good to inject directly into your blood stream without negative consequences to your health. One read of *Miller's Review of Critical Vaccine Studies* or one watch of any of Gary Null's vaccine documentaries and you will probably be in tears over how horrific vaccines really are. Even if they are good for you, shouldn't you have a choice about what is injected into your own body? Meanwhile, Bill Gates' money has been responsible for injecting these gruesome ingredients into 760 million children around the world and the vaccination mandates are presently being planned in California and New York to take away your choice, under the influence of none other than Bill Gates, along with other players of course. To each their own, again, each person's situation is different. If you decide to get vaccinated that is your prerogative. Again, I am only defending having a choice over the matter. But vaccines are a HUGE subject for another article. Anyway, here's a little more on William. His numerous grants have granted him a huge influence on the policies that the CDC and WHO put forward. These are not the only agencies Bill Gates has under his thumb either. You better believe it, he has slowly but surely monopolized global, public health through various charitable donations and stock options. Let's remember also, Bill Gates became one of the richest men in the world by creating Microsoft Windows, which was made with an operating system **pirated** from Gary Kildall and Xerox, not entirely of his own creation, he was **sued** by the U.S. government in the 90s prior to his release of Microsoft Windows '98, and **Bill Gates is not a doctor, an epidemiologist, or a certified infectious disease researcher**. And let's not forget that **The Bill and Melinda Gates Foundation is a major funding source for the Pirbright Institute, proud owner of U.S. patent number 10,130,701 B2, a patent approved in 2018 on a coronavirus vaccine**. You think the vaccine will really take a year to develop as you were originally told? Think again. Maybe that's just what they wanted you to believe. My guess is that Bill stands to make a lot of bills by telling us that everyone needs to be vaccinated. By the way, he has also called for a national tracking system to be put in place to know who has COVID-19 and who has or hasn't been vaccinated and his money is already working on giving people quantum dot tattoos for this purpose. Plus, Microsoft, in alliance with Accenture, IDEO, Gavi, and the Rockefeller Foundation and supported by the U.N. is working on ID2020, which may seek to use RFID microchip implants to be able to digitally identify everyone and track them. Then in October/November of 2019, Bill's foundation put on a pandemic "exercise" that "simulated" a major coronavirus outbreak one month **prior** to when the actual coronavirus outbreak occurred in December of 2019 called **Event 201**. At this round-table sat representatives from Johnson and Johnson, Johns Hopkins University, **China CDC**, Bill and Melinda Gates Foundation, ANZ Bank Group, UPS Foundation, UN, Former US Deputy National Security Advisor, US CDC, World Bank Group, and NBC Universal. If you watched this event, as I did, you would have seen that companies were basically jockeying for position, persuading, and promoting the need of the private sector to respond to such a pandemic to get their share of the profits from such a "potential" outbreak. You would also notice how the U.S. CDC representative is wearing a military uniform (maybe the man is ex military) and says, "Governments are going to need to be willing to do things that are out of their historical perspective. For the most part it's really a **war footing** that we need to be on". Another participant from Henry Schein says we need to escalate entrepreneurship and have subsidies and tax breaks given to companies from the government so they can make more products and advocates for a "**MARTIAL type plan**". Martial law anyone? A participant from Edelman basically says that social media platforms need to **censor** misinformation and change their position from being technology platforms to broadcasters and that they need to partner with scientific and health communities to "flood the zone" with "accurate" information. A rep of the Monetary Authority of Singapore wonders if governments should step up their efforts on "enforcement actions against fake news". Bye bye net neutrality. Remember, this event was held BEFORE any public knowledge of any actual pandemic. And what happened a few months later after Event 201 when we were in real, full pandemic mode? The dominoes fell exactly like these people planned. I was personally censored a number of times for my truth-telling Facebook posts, and other "in the know" videos continue to disappear from YouTube daily. What's more, in 2010 **Gates bought 500,000 shares of GMO giant Monsanto** valued at $23 million, Gates' father was on the board of Planned Parenthood, which was birthed out of the **American Eugenics Society**, and, recently, Bill Gates stepped down from being on the board of directors for **Berkshire Hathaway**, the owner of Acme Bricks, the company that allegedly delivered loads of bricks to major cities around the country at the height of the George Floyd protests. This last one is off topic, I know, but is it really? Just continuing the Bill Gates onslaught here, sorry. Another fact of the matter is that **all of these agencies/companies/individuals generally follow the Big Pharma, allopathic, standard of care, conventional, medical model and generally do not acknowledge alternative medicine nor the natural health industry and often go so far as to call it's remedies, some of which have hundreds of thousands of studies on them and a 5,000 year track record of use, safety, and efficacy, far longer than any such invention as synthetic**

pharmaceutical drugs and vaccines, quackery. And maybe Gates and his CDC have good intentions, maybe Gates believes what he is doing is right, maybe he believes he is improving peoples' health and when you improve peoples' health then they choose to have less kids because they know those kids are more likely to survive, thus justifying the depopulation agenda he admits to in numerous interviews and TED talks. If so, if he thinks he is helping people with all of his "philanthropy" and if he isn't intentionally doing evil, well then that's only because he's a civilized, westernized, modernist and technologist, not a naturopath or naturalist. Maybe it's just ignorance on his part. Maybe it's just completely unbeknownst to him that **modern technology does not give health. Nature gives health. Nature *is* health. And health *is* nature. Health only comes from nature. It has always been so, and will always be so. Anything that is unnatural and does not obey nature's laws always has a side effect and negative consequence.** And maybe we do need to reduce population, but vaccination and GMOs and Planned Parenthood's recommendation that fibroid causing, cancer causing birth control is a "safe and easy way to prevent pregnancy" is not the way to go. Maybe it would be better if we just used our resources more wisely and frugally and funded solar and wind power and electric cars and changed monocrop GMO farming to permaculture farming and offered incentives for having less children and improved family planning education or some other wiser, healthier, more natural method. But enough about all of that. I had to unmask some of the parties involved, though, in this masked debate about face masks, to have an honest conversation about it and provide some context for this proceeding. So, on account of the reasons above, **I think the answer as to whether these agencies and individuals can be trusted to provide the right information as regards our health or not, is probably no**. But I am not the doctor here. Once again, legally I must say that you should probably hear out your government and your doctor before making any decisions. But I didn't even get into **Anthony Fauci** or any of the other goons on the tube telling you what to do. A simple viewing of part 1 of the "Plandemic" documentary will suffice for his indictment, that is, if you can find it, since all major search engines have censored and buried it. I'll give you a little teaser though, Fauci is the director of the National Institute of Allergy and Infectious Diseases which, prior to the pandemic gave $7.4 million to the Wuhan Institute of Virology lab in Wuhan, China that was studying coronaviruses in bats and also, **Fauci owns** multiple patents, one of which is **patent number US20030180254A1, a patent on IL-2 therapy, which is the therapy that he, along with Robert Redfield, current director of the CDC, directed AIDS patients receive during that pandemic back in the 80s, allegedly after 2 years of holding up the confirmation of the virus until the patents were pushed through.** Again, I'm not claiming there's some massive organized conspiracy and that these people and agencies are doing these things with nefarious intentions, it might just be ignorance or power hunger, or in the case of Fauci greed and ignorance, and they might just be caught up in the same modern machine we are all caught up in that we just can't seem to stop or escape from. Alright alright. Sorry. That's enough for now. The rabbit hole is just so deep I couldn't help myself. Now the stage is set to present some real information on respirators and face masks, not opinion and not conjecture nor secondhand hearsay.

Firstly, what are the **differences** between **respirators** and **surgical masks**? It is important to distinguish the two when interpreting their effectiveness. The **CDC** and the **CCHOS** states that respirators, such as the **N95** mask, are evaluated, tested, and approved by the **National Institute for Occupational Safety and Healthcare** and are **said** to protect against airborne particles and biological aerosols such as **bacteria and viruses**. Surgical masks, on the other hand, are cleared by the Food and Drug Administration and act simply as a barrier to splashes, droplets, spit, and other hazardous fluids. **Respirators** are said to reduce the **wearer's exposure** to particles, while **surgical masks** are **said** to protect **other people** from the wearer's respiratory emissions. Respirators are tight fitting and are generally single use but may be used more than once, surgical masks are not tight fitting and they are for single use only (one patient encounter). **According to the CDC, surgical masks do NOT protect**

the wearer from inhaling airborne particles such as pathogens.

However, other than just listening to these governing bodies, since I have already exposed their conflicts of interest, lets look at some **scientific studies** to determine if masks are even effective at all. When interpreting medical journal studies, just like interpreting whether the CDC or WHO are trustworthy, it can be consequential to consider if there are **conflicts of interest** inherent in such studies. For example, a study showing that secondhand smoke is NOT harmful, funded by a tobacco company, just might be a little bit biased, because it benefits the company's bottom line to show a favorable outcome. I did not see any major conflicts of interest declared in the studies below, but that doesn't mean they don't exist. In the example of scientific reviews published in journals on secondhand smoke, one study showed that 77% of the authors of the reviews did not disclose their sources of funding[2]. Furthermore, Richard Horton, editor of The Lancet (a peer-reviewed medical journal) stated that **perhaps half of scientific literature in general may simply be untrue** do to conflicts of interest and other problems.[3] Nevertheless, taken with a grain of salt, here we go...

Scientific Studies on Respirator/Mask-Wearing

Ann Intern Med 2020: "Neither surgical nor cotton masks effectively filtered SARS–CoV-2 during coughs by infected patients. Prior evidence that surgical masks effectively filtered influenza virus (1) informed recommendations that patients with confirmed or suspected COVID-19 should wear face masks to prevent transmission (2)."[4] "Oberg and Brousseau (3) demonstrated that **surgical masks did not exhibit adequate filter performance** against aerosols measuring 0.9, 2.0, and 3.1 µm in diameter. Lee and colleagues (4) showed that **particles 0.04 to 0.2 µm can penetrate surgical masks**. The size of the SARS–CoV particle from the 2002–2004 outbreak was estimated as 0.08 to 0.14 µm (5); assuming that SARS-CoV-2 has a similar size, **surgical masks are unlikely to effectively filter this virus."[3] "This experiment did not include N95 masks".[4]**

elife 2020: "Measurements of the particle filtration efficiency of N95 masks show that they are capable of filtering ≈99.8% of particles with a diameter of ≈0.1 µm [100-120 nm] (Rengasamy et al., 2017). **SARS-CoV-2 is an enveloped virus ≈0.1 µm in diameter, so N95 masks are capable of filtering most free virions**, but they do more than that. How so? Viruses are often transmitted through respiratory droplets produced by coughing and sneezing."[5] "The characteristic diameter of large droplets produced by sneezing is ~100 µm (Han et al., 2013), while the diameter of droplet nuclei produced by coughing is on the order of ~1 µm (Yang et al., 2007). At present, it is unclear whether surfaces or air are the dominant mode of SARS-CoV-2 transmission, but N95 masks should provide some protection against both (Jefferson et al., 2009; Leung et al., 2020)."[5]

ACS Nano 2020 Study: "Although the filtration efficiencies for various fabrics when a single layer was used ranged from 5 to 80% and 5 to 95% for particle sizes of <300 nm and >300 nm, respectively, the efficiencies improved when multiple layers were used and when using a specific combination of different fabrics. Filtration efficiencies of the hybrids (such as cotton-silk, cotton-chiffon, cotton-flannel) was >80% (for particles <300 nm) and >90% (for particles >300 nm). We speculate that the **enhanced performance of the hybrids** is likely due to the combined effect of mechanical and electrostatic-based filtration. **Cotton,** the most widely used material for cloth masks **performs better at higher weave densities** (i.e., thread count) and can make a significant difference in filtration efficiencies. Our studies also imply that gaps (as caused by an **improper fit of the mask) can result in over a 60% decrease in the filtration** efficiency, implying the need for future cloth mask design studies to take into account issues of "fit" and leakage, while allowing the exhaled air to vent efficiently. Overall, we find that combinations of various commonly available fabrics used in **cloth masks can potentially provide significant protection against the transmission of aerosol particles.**"[6]

BMJ 2020: "That trial, which was considered robust, **showed a benefit of masks over no masks, but no benefit of respirator masks over standard ones**, and also showed that masks were worn less than 50% of the time".[7]

"A 2010 systematic review of face masks in influenza epidemics, which included standard surgical masks and respirator masks and **found some efficacy of masks if worn by those with respiratory symptoms but not if worn by asymptomatic individuals.**"[7]

"A 2007 systematic review and expert panel deliberation, which acknowledged the difficulties in interpreting evidence and stated: "**With the exception of some evidence from SARS, we did not find any published data that directly support the use of masks … by the public.**""[7]

"Xiao and colleagues reviewed non-pharmaceutical measures for prevention of influenza. They identified 10 randomised controlled trials published between 1946 and 2018 that tested the efficacy of face masks (including standard surgical masks and commercially produced paper face masks designed for the public) for preventing laboratory confirmed influenza. A pooled meta-analysis **found no significant reduction in influenza transmission** (relative risk 0.78, 95% confidence interval 0.51 to 1.20; I2=30%, P=0.25). They also identified seven studies conducted in households; four provided masks for all household members, one for the sick member only, and two for household contacts only. **None showed a significant reduction in laboratory confirmed influenza in the face mask arm**. The authors concluded: "**randomized controlled trials of [face masks] did not support a substantial effect on transmission of laboratory-confirmed influenza.**""[7]

"A...systematic review published on 6 April 2020 examined whether wearing a face mask or other barrier (goggles, shield, veil) prevents transmission of respiratory illness such as coronavirus, rhinovirus, tuberculosis, or influenza. It identified 31 eligible studies, including 12 randomised controlled trials. The authors found that overall, **mask wearing both in general and by infected members within households seemed to produce small but statistically non-significant reductions in infection rates**. The authors concluded that "**The evidence is not sufficiently strong to support the widespread use of facemasks as a protective measure against covid-19** and recommended further high quality randomised controlled trials."[7]

PLOS ONE 2008 Study: "Any type of general mask use is **likely to decrease viral exposure and infection risk** on a population level, in spite of imperfect fit and imperfect adherence, personal respirators providing most protection. Masks worn by patients may not offer as great a degree of protection against aerosol transmission."[8]

BMC Public Health 2007: "Other non-pharmaceutical interventions including **mask-use and other personal protective equipment for the general public, school and workplace closures early in an epidemic, and mandatory travel restrictions were rejected as likely to be ineffective, infeasible, or unacceptable to the public.**"[9]

AM J Infect Control. 2009: "**Face mask use in health care workers has not been demonstrated to provide benefit in terms of cold symptoms or getting colds**. A larger study is needed to definitively establish noninferiority of no mask use."[10]

Epidemiol. Infect. 2010: "**Wearing masks incorrectly may increase the risk of transmission.**"

"While there is some experimental evidence that masks should be able to reduce infectiousness under controlled conditions, there is less evidence on whether this translates to effectiveness in natural settings. **There is little evidence to support the effectiveness of face masks to reduce the risk of infection.**"[11]

Influenza and Other Respiratory Viruses 2011: "**...one trial found a lower rate of clinical respiratory illness associated with the use of non-fit-tested N95 respirators compared with medical masks, whilst a non-inferiority trial found that masks and respirators offered similar protection** to nurses against laboratory-confirmed influenza infection. A trial conducted amongst crowded, urban households found that, despite poor compliance, **mask wearing coupled with hand sanitizer use, reduced secondary transmission of upper respiratory infection/influenza-like illness/laboratory-confirmed influenza compared with education; hand sanitizer alone resulted in no reduction** in this aggregated outcome. Although **the remaining five trials found no significant differences** between control and intervention groups, there were some notable findings. **Household contacts who wore a P2 respirator** (considered to have an equivalent rating to an N95 respirator) **'all' or 'most' of the time for the first days were less likely to develop an influenza-like illness compared with less frequent users in one study.**"[12]

J Evid Based Med. 2020: "This meta-analysis showed that **there were no statistically significant differences in preventing laboratory-confirmed influenza, laboratory-confirmed respiratory viral infections, laboratory-confirmed res-piratory infection and influenza-like illness using N95 respirators and surgical masks**. N95 respirators provided a protective effect against laboratory-confirmed bacterial colonization."[13]

JAMA 2019: "This supports the finding that **neither N95 respirators nor medical masks were more effective in preventing laboratory-confirmed influenza or other viral respiratory infection or illness among participants when worn in a fashion consistent with current US clinical practice.**"[14]

Other Considerations

Okay. We know some differences now between types of face masks and we've seen that **the studies on respirators/masks show mixed results as to whether they work or not.** So it seems we are back to square one. Well, not exactly, because **there are many other things to think about when determining whether one should wear a mask** besides whether or not they filter viruses and/or reduce the transmission of respiratory influenza-like illnesses. For example, the Health and Safety Practices Survey of Healthcare Workers on the CDC website recommends that all workers required to wear a tight fitting respirator **have a medical evaluation to determine whether they are capable of wearing one.** Though I've maligned the CDC and the WHO, not everything they say is entirely wrong, the sentiment of some of what they say is correct and/or a good idea. I'm not saying you should go have a "medical" evaluation to determine if you are capable of wearing one, but you may want to think twice about it and, along with your practitioner, determine for yourself whether you think you are capable of wearing one. So, one question to ask yourself is, am I healthy enough to wear a mask to begin with? One should also consider that **a person aged 40-49 is probably more likely to die from car accidents, falling, MRSA, accidental poisoning, suicide, flu, hospital infections, stroke, cancer, and heart disease than from COVID-19.**[15,16] If you are aged 40 - 49, and driving your car and going to the hospital may be more hazardous than corona, then why the big hubbub about it? Because the media chooses what it wants to focus on. On that note, I'm sure some of us have heard about the man who died in a car wreck after passing out from wearing a mask because it restricted his oxygen intake and caused a build up of carbon dioxide in his body. Therefore, we should also inquire - **does excess CO_2 build up inside masks and is excess CO_2 bad for you? Yes, CO_2 does build up in N95 masks**, as shown by a study from 2010, published in the journal Respiratory Care.[17] And yes, **excess CO_2 is bad for you**. It is a known toxicant, can effect cognitive performance, decision making, problem resolution, cause unconsciousness, **respiratory symptoms, and respiratory arrest!**[18,19] The very things you're trying to prevent from happening from COVID! Moreover, wearing a face mask while driving, obviously increases the already higher risk of dying from driving versus COVID! **Enclosed environments are more vulnerable to CO_2 buildup** too! And what are we all being told to do? Stay inside! Stay inside your car and stay inside your homes! Meanwhile, **CO_2 levels have been rising on the planet for decades** also! At the same time all of this is going on, **5G** is being installed everywhere in America and studies have shown many harmful effects (Kostoff, 2019) and that oxygen absorbs the 60GHz frequency (Tretyakov, 2005), which may be employed in the future of 5G, so people have theorized that this **may prevent hemoglobin from effectively binding with oxygen** (plus the book *The Invisible Rainbow: A History of Electricity and Life* correlates that the occurrence of epidemics/pandemics often come soon after large scale new electrical devices/networks have been set up on Earth). To put a cherry on top of the mounds of evidence here and the heaps of mask cream piling up at landfills and polluting the planet everywhere, **one of the major complications that leads to a person's death from COVID-19 is hypoxia** (a lack of oxygen because the lungs fill up with fluid) (Huang, 2020). It sure sounds like there's a giant conspiracy to induce hypoxic hysteria on the masses to me. I might die of irony overload writing this, or perhaps all the iron I'm accumulating will save me by building more red blood cells to carry more oxygen in my body. Or, I could just not wear a mask, wear some EMF blocking clothing, take some natural dietary supplements, and eat healthily and maybe I'll be spared of the perilous plague possibly perpetrated upon us! Whew! I'm a little out of breath now after all that. Anyway, jokes aside, if the man who died in the car wreck's family members are aware of these facts, the irony of them in relation to the tragic fate of the man, they are likely to be haunted and guilt-ridden by them forever. Not to mention, **the number of cases of COVID-19 and the death rates from COVID-19 are inflated** anyway due to the fact that some of the tests do not actually test for the SARS-CoV-2 virus, the virus that causes COVID-19, and due to the fact that they are classifying deaths as COVID-19 deaths if a person came into contact with somebody who had COVID-19, but did not necessarily die from COVID-19. As Deborah Birx, one of the physicians leading the White House's Coronavirus Task Force said, "We've taken a very liberal approach to mortality". **Coronaviruses are among the most frequent causes of the common cold** (Paules et al.). What else should we take into account about masks? Well, it turns out there are other detrimental health effects of wearing them. One study showed an **increase in headaches** of participants wearing masks.[10] Another showed a potential for development of **skin lesions, irritant dermatitis, or worsening acne** when used frequently for long hours.[20] There's a **potential increased risk of self-contamination due to the manipulation of a face mask**.[21, 22] Difficulty breathing and tiredness may be caused by mask-wearing (Kim et al.), (Esposito et al.). And **what about inhaling bleach**? The CDC recommends either washing face masks in your washing machine with your other laundry or hand washing them with bleach. The WHO recommends pretty much the same thing but says when you can't use hot water, then either boil the mask or use .1% chlorine then thoroughly rinse the mask afterward. If one doesn't have hot water or a washing machine, then one ought to ask themselves, **which is more risky, the possibility of catching coronavirus, or inhaling chlorine bleach every day for the past 6 months that this virus has been around and well into the future?** "Chlorine gas is a potent pulmonary irritant that causes acute damage in both the upper and lower respiratory tract."[23] Still, there's more. **Should the same face mask recommendations be given across the board depending on the state one lives in? Does one's blood type reduce their risk of infection? What affect does temperature and humidity have on the** coronavirus? What other precautionary measures is a person taking besides wearing a mask? **Are masks and hand sanitizers the only way to protect oneself from infection and complications from infection? Are they the best ways? Is one weakening one's immune system by filtering out healthy bacteria and viruses in the air? Does relying solely on a mask and hand sanitizer give a person a false sense of security that leads them to not take other more important precautionary measures against the virus?** Let's answer these questions too. **In Florida, we live in a very hot and humid state**. Preliminary evidence published in 2020 showed that **higher temperatures are associated with lower incidence of COVID-19**.[24] In March, Live Science posted an article that stated that 90% of Coronavirus infections occurred in areas between 37.4 and 62.6 degrees Fahrenheit. Less than 6% of global cases occurred in countries with an average temperature above 64.4 degrees and an absolute humidity above 9 g/m3. Some researchers have gone so far as to propose a weather pattern that COVID-19 follows along called the Corona Belt. Influenza is always more prominent in the winter-time due to drier and colder weather. Shaman et al. demonstrated in a study[25] from 2010 that absolute **humidity is likely the predominant determinant of influenza seasonality**. There are other sides to this coin, though. Florida was ranked 18th in the country for per capita (per 100 people) COVID cases as of April, 2020 and 19th in case fatality rate in May, 2020. Not great, but not terrible either. But, we do have a lot of old people. The state rankings you see on T.V. are not usually per capita, just the amount of cases for the whole state. Some states are bigger than others. Does blood type increase or decrease one's risk of COVID-19? A non peer-reviewed pre-print of a study from 2020 showed that blood group A is associated with an increased risk of COVID-19 and blood group O is associated with a decreased risk (Zhao, 2020). Roughly 40% of Americans have type O blood. What other measures is a person or business taking besides wearing or mandating masks to employees and are they better than masks? **Some health food stores run an ozonator daily** to purify the air. Ozone is an eco-friendly, yet powerful trioxygen disinfectant that is produced naturally within Earth's atmosphere. It can oxidize anything including viruses, bacteria, and organic and inorganic molecules. Some health food stores know to tightly control the levels of ozone in the store to purify the air in a safe and healthy fashion. Some retail vitamin shops are in the process of installing **UV light** within their air conditioning system to purify the air. Nearly all stores currently offer **curbside service** for those who do not wish to go inside. Some health food stores use tiny amounts of hydrogen peroxide in their cleaning solution and **sanitize carts and baskets at the front door. 6 foot social distancing measures are in place** with floor markings at most businesses. At this time, many stores are making it **mandatory for at least a portion of their employees to wear masks** as well. And, last but not least, if you shop at a local health food store for your groceries and natural medicine, then you may be taking less of a risk than shopping at some big box store. This is because the other customers who shop at a health food store are likely eating healthily and taking natural immune boosting supplements, possibly reducing the chances of infection and the spreading germs. For example, olive leaf extract has been shown to reduce viral shedding (Renis et al., Micol et al.). I think we've answered a few questions with those last sentences but I can't answer them all. But lets ask some more shall we!? Questioning the allopathic, conventional, big pharma, medical model recommendations and the mainstream media's narrative is, after all, probably one of the healthiest things we can do when it comes to this "pandemic". Some of the questions below are borrowed from an article by Denis G. Rancourt, PhD.

Unknown Aspects and Unanswered Questions of Mask-Wearing:

Does a community of natural health-minded people have the same risk for the spread of infection as the general public?
Should the government be in charge of your health or you?

Do used masks become sources of enhanced transmission, for the wearer and others?
Do masks collect and retain pathogens that the mask wearer would otherwise avoid when breathing naturally without a mask?
Are large droplets caught by a mask atomized or aerosolized into inhalable components?
Can virions escape an evaporating droplet stuck to a face mask?
What are the dangers of bacterial growth on a used mask?
How do pathogen-laden droplets interact with other environmental particles captured on the mask?
What are the long-term health effects of impeded breathing?
Are there negative social consequences to a masked society?
Are there negative psychological consequences to wearing a mask, as a fear-based behavioral modification?
What are the environmental consequences of mask manufacturing and disposal?
Do the masks shed fibres or substances that are harmful when inhaled?'

Summary: What Have We Learned?

- Wearing or not wearing a mask is a personal choice and nobody should be shamed for making either choice

- Government agencies claim that N95 respirators are different than surgical masks and claim that they offer more protection for the wearer against viruses

- Surgical masks are for single, one patient/person encounter use only and are only claimed to offer minor protection for other people of one's respiratory emissions and are not claimed to protect a wearer against viruses

- Some studies show that respirators/masks work and some studies show they don't work

- Respirators might work better than surgical masks or not or neither of them work

- An improperly fitted mask may increase the risk of transmission or it may not

- Half of the scientific literature may be fraudulent

- The science is NEVER settled

- Bill Gates has given the CDC and WHO a lot of money which may cause conflicts of interest in their recommendations

- Getting vaccinated with a flu vaccine may possibly increase one's risk of being infected with coronaviruses and vaccines may not be healthy for you

- A simulated coronavirus outbreak called Event 201 was staged and funded by The Bill and Melinda Gates Foundation roughly one month prior to the actual outbreak

- Pandemics/epidemics may possibly coincide with new large scale electromagnetic devices/networks being set up on Earth

- One may need to have a medical evaluation to determine if one is healthy enough to wear a mask

- A person aged 40-49 is more likely to die from car accidents, falling, MRSA, accidental poisoning, suicide, flu, hospital infections, stroke, cancer, and heart disease than from COVID-19

- COVID-19 death rates are inflated

- Coronaviruses are among the most frequent causes of the common cold

- Florida is a hot, humid state and higher temps and higher humidity is associated with less incidence of COVID-19

- Blood type may play a role in one's risk of contracting COVID-19

- There are other precautions one can take to bolster one's health besides mask-wearing

- Some health food stores purify their air with ozone

- Some vitamin shops are installing UV light in their A/C system to kill pathogens

- Some health food stores disinfect carts and baskets

- Many businesses apply social distancing measures with floor markings

- Many stores already make it mandatory for at least a portion of their employees to wear masks

- Health food stores sell antiviral dietary supplements and healthy food

- **There are detrimental health consequences of wearing masks such as:**

- Difficulty breathing

- Increased headaches

- Elevated CO_2 levels

- Maybe more likely to die in a car while wearing a mask

- Inhaling of toxic bleach

- Skin lesions, irritant dermatitis, or worsening acne has been documented in studies on wearing masks

- Potential increased risk of self-contamination from wearing a mask

- Tiredness

- The jury is still out as to whether masks work or not and blindly accepting that they work may put one more at risk due to having a false sense of security, while not taking other important precautions

- There are unanswered questions if masks have other detrimental effects

- It is probably healthy to question the allopathic, conventional, medical model recommendations and the mainstream media's narrative and stance on masks, but you should always talk to your doctor/naturopath/practitioner before making any changes/decisions

Hopefully all of this information I have presented you with puts your mind and lungs at ease when going out in public. I appreciate your patronage and believe that I am going above and beyond and taking more than adequate precautionary measures to ensure the safety and health of myself and others. You are responsible for your own health and your own decisions. I am not liable whether you choose to wear a mask or not. I only present information for your consideration. You should always talk to your doctor or holistic practitioner before making any changes. If you have other questions about what you can do to support your immune system in this challenging time, I have other protocols I have created that are either free or available for purchase on my website and I am equipped with the skill and knowledge to assist you in a consultation if you would like one. Breathe easy.

References:
1. Wolff GG. Influenza vaccination and respiratory virus interference among Department of Defense personnel during the 2017-2018 influenza season. Vaccine. 2020;38(2):350-354. doi:10.1016/j.vaccine.2019.10.005
2. Barnes DE, Bero LA. Why review articles on the health effects of passive smoking reach different conclusions. JAMA. 1998;279(19):1566-1570. doi:10.1001/jama.279.19.1566
3. Gyles C. Skeptical of medical science reports?. Can Vet J. 2015;56(10):1011-1012.
4. Bae S, Kim MC, Kim JY, et al. Effectiveness of Surgical and Cotton Masks in Blocking SARS-CoV-2: A Controlled Comparison in 4 Patients [published online ahead of print, 2020 Apr 6] [retracted in: Ann Intern Med. 2020 Jun 2;:]. Ann Intern Med. 2020;M20-1342. doi:10.7326/M20-1342
5. Bar-On YM, Flamholz A, Phillips R, Milo R. SARS-CoV-2 (COVID-19) by the numbers. Elife. 2020;9:e57309. Published 2020 Apr 2. doi:10.7554/eLife.57309
6. Konda A, Prakash A, Moss GA, Schmoldt M, Grant GD, Guha S. Aerosol Filtration Efficiency of Common Fabrics Used in Respiratory Cloth Masks. ACS Nano. 2020;14(5):6339-6347. doi:10.1021/acsnano.0c03252
7. Greenhalgh Trisha, Schmid Manuel B, Czypionka Thomas, Bassler Dirk, Gruer Laurence. Face masks for the public during the covid-19 crisis BMJ 2020; 369 :m1435
8. van der Sande M, Teunis P, Sabel R. Professional and home-made face masks reduce exposure to respiratory infections among the general population. PLoS One. 2008;3(7):e2618. Published 2008 Jul 9. doi:10.1371/journal.pone.0002618
9. Aledort JE, Lurie N, Wasserman J, Bozzette SA. Non-pharmaceutical public health interventions for

pandemic influenza: an evaluation of the evidence base. BMC Public Health. 2007;7:208. Published 2007 Aug 15. doi:10.1186/1471-2458-7-208

10. Jacobs JL, Ohde S, Takahashi O, Tokuda Y, Omata F, Fukui T. Use of surgical face masks to reduce the incidence of the common cold among health care workers in Japan: a randomized controlled trial. Am J Infect Control. 2009;37(5):417-419. doi:10.1016/j.ajic.2008.11.002

11. COWLING, B. J., ZHOU, Y., IP, D. K. M., LEUNG, G. M., & AIELLO, A. E. (2010). Face masks to prevent transmission of influenza virus: a systematic review. Epidemiology and Infection, 138(04), 449. doi:10.1017/s0950268809991658

12. Bin-Reza, Faisal & Lopez Chavarrias, Vicente & Nicoll, Angus & Chamberland, Mary. (2011). The use of masks and respirators to prevent transmission of influenza: A systematic review of the scientific evidence. Influenza and other respiratory viruses. 6. 257-67. 10.1111/j.1750-2659.2011.00307.x.

13. Long Y, Hu T, Liu L, et al. Effectiveness of N95 respirators versus surgical masks against influenza: A systematic review and meta-analysis. J Evid Based Med. 2020;13(2):93-101. doi:10.1111/jebm.12381

14. Radonovich LJ Jr, Simberkoff MS, Bessesen MT, et al. N95 Respirators vs Medical Masks for Preventing Influenza Among Health Care Personnel: A Randomized Clinical Trial. JAMA. 2019;322(9):824-833. doi:10.1001/jama.2019.11645

15. All accidental death information from National Safety Council. Disease death information from Centers for Disease Control and Prevention. Shark fatality data provided by the International Shark Attack File. Lifetime risk is calculated by dividing 2003 population (290,850,005) by the number of deaths, divided by 77.6, the life expectancy of a person born in 2003.

16. The Epidemiological Characteristics of an Outbreak of 2019 Novel Coronavirus Diseases (COVID-19) - China CCDC, February 17 2020. Report of the WHO-China Joint Mission on Coronavirus Disease 2019 (COVID-19) [Pdf] - World Health Organization, Feb. 28, 2020.

17. Roberge RJ, Coca A, Williams WJ, Powell JB, Palmiero AJ. Physiological impact of the N95 filtering facepiece respirator on healthcare workers. Respir Care. 2010;55(5):569-577.

18. Azuma, K., Kagi, N., Yanagi, U., & Osawa, H. (2018). Effects of low-level inhalation exposure to carbon dioxide in indoor environments: A short review on human health and psychomotor performance. Environment International, 121, 51–56. doi:10.1016/j.envint.2018.08.059

19. Permentier K, Vercammen S, Soetaert S, Schellemans C. Carbon dioxide poisoning: a literature review of an often forgotten cause of intoxication in the emergency department. Int J Emerg Med. 2017;10(1):14. doi:10.1186/s12245-017-0142-y

20. Al Badri F. Surgical mask contact dermatitis and epidemiology of contact dermatitis in healthcare workers. . Current Allergy & Clinical Immunology, 30,3: 183 - 188. 2017.

21. Zamora JE, Murdoch J, Simchison B, Day AG. Contamination: a comparison of 2 personal protective systems. CMAJ. 2006;175(3):249-54.

22. Kwon JH, Burnham CD, Reske KA, Liang SY, Hink T, Wallace MA, et al. Assessment of Healthcare Worker Protocol Deviations and Self-Contamination During Personal Protective Equipment Donning and Doffing. Infect Control Hosp Epidemiol. 2017;38(9):1077-83.

23. Akdur O, Durukan P, Ikizceli I, Ozkan S, Avsarogullari L. A rare complication of chlorine gas inhalation: pneumomediastinum. Emerg Med J. 2006;23(11):e59. doi:10.1136/emj.2006.040022

24. Bannister-Tyrrell, Melanie & Meyer, Anne & Faverjon, Céline & Cameron, Angus. (2020). Preliminary evidence that higher temperatures are associated with lower incidence of COVID-19, for cases reported globally up to 29th February 2020. 10.1101/2020.03.18.20036731.

25. Shaman J, Pitzer VE, Viboud C, Grenfell BT, Lipsitch M. Absolute humidity and the seasonal onset of influenza in the continental United States [published correction appears in PLoS Biol. 2010;8(3). doi: 10.1371/annotation/35686514-b7a9-4f65-9663-7baefc0d63c0]. PLoS Biol. 2010;8(2):e1000316. Published 2010 Feb 23. doi:10.1371/journal.pbio.1000316

Vaccine Information Resources

Collin Gow, C.N.C.

Documentaries

1. The Silent Epidemic: The Untold Story of Vaccines (2013) (Gary Null, Ph.D.)
2. Vaccine Nation (2008) (Gary Null, Ph.D.)
3. The Quiet Killer - The Exploding Autoimmune Epidemics – Vaccines and Man Made Cancer – Dr. Randy Tent (Dr. Randy Tent)
4. Death By Medicine (2011) (Gary Null, Ph.D.)
5. Shots in the Dark: Silence on Vaccine (2009) (Lina B. Moreco)
6. Vaxxed: From Cover-up to Catastrophe (2016) (Dr. Andrew Wakefield)
7. Vaccination: The Hidden Truth (1998)
8. Hear the Silence (2003) (Dr. Andrew Wakefield)
9. Autism: Made in the USA (2009) (Gary Null, Ph.D.)
10. Deadly Deception (Gary Null Ph.D.)
11. In Lies We Trust – The CIA, Hollywood, and Bioterrorism (Leonard G. Horowitz)

Books

1. Miller's Review of Critical Vaccine Studies: 400 Important Scientific Papers Summarized for Parents and Researchers (2016) (Neil Z. Miller)
2. Dr. Mary's Monkey (2015) (Edward T. Haslam)
3. Thimerosal: Let the Science Speak: The Evidence Supporting the Immediate Removal of Mercury–a Known Neurotoxin–from Vaccines (2014) (Robert F. Kennedy Jr.)
4. Death By Medicine (2010) (Gary Null, Ph.D.)
5. Emerging Viruses – AIDS and Ebola (1996) (Leonard G. Horowitz)

Vaccine Ingredients

https://www.cdc.gov/vaccines/pubs/pinkbook/downloads/appendices/b/excipient-table-2.pdf

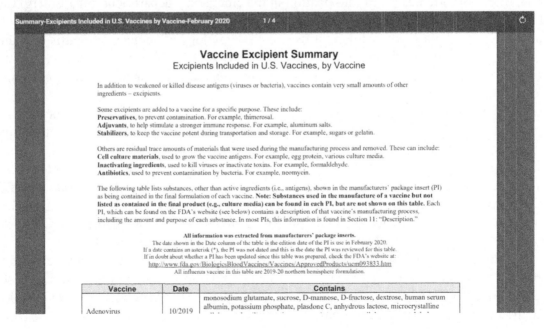

Toxic Vaccine Excipients and Their Effects

By Collin Gow, C.N.C.

11/24/2020

MRC-5: human fetal lung fibroblast cells originally derived from a 14 week old male fetus aborted in 1966. In an open letter to legislators regarding fetal cell DNA in vaccines, Dr. Theresa Deisher wrote that human fetal DNA contaminates vaccines and can reach a blood level in a vaccinated child that is known to activate TLR9, which can cause autoimmune attacks. Non-self DNA may cross react with a child's own DNA, according to Deisher. Children with autism have antibodies against human DNA in their circulation and increased levels of autism corresponded to the introduction of and/or increased doses of MMR, varicella, and hepatitis A vaccines containing fetal DNA (Deisher et al.) (https://www.soundchoice.org/open-letter-to-legislators/). Dr. Helen Ratajczak has suggested an increased prevalence of autism from human DNA being added to vaccines too. Also, an increased spike in autism has been documented since the chicken pox virus began being cultured in human fetal tissue for vaccines in 1995 (Ratajczak et al.).

Vero cells: monkey kidney cells which may be contaminated with other pathogenic microbes not intended to be in the vaccine (Osada et al.) (Vilchez et al.).

Human serum albumin: protein from human blood.

Calf bovine serum albumin: protein from the blood of baby cows. A study published in the New England Journal of Medicine found that bovine serum albumin causes membranous nephropathy in early childhood (Debiec et al.).

CRM 197 carrier protein: "non-toxic" mutant of diphtheria toxin, yet some studies have shown it to be toxic to yeast cells and mammalian cells (Kimura et al.). "Functions as a carrier for polysaccharides and haptens, making them immunogenic."

Plasdone C: pyrogen free water-soluble adhesive/polymer.

Anhydrous lactose: water-free milk sugar.

Polacrilin potassium: weakly acidic cation exchange resin/plastic.

Cellulose acetate phthalate: compound consisting of a polysaccharide, often from the cell walls of plants, as well as acetic acid, and an ester of phthalic anhydride. Phthalates are endocrine disrupting plasticizer chemicals banned in some children's toys and banned in cosmetics and personal care products in California and Europe. They may cause rhinitis, eczema, asthma, reduced penile size, incomplete testicular descent, and other issues (Meeker et al.).

Acetone: flammable organic solvent used in nail polish and paint thinner.

FD&C Yellow #6 aluminum lake dye: artificial color shown to cause hypersensitivity reactions

(Kobylewski et al.), allergic reactions (EFSA, 2009), attention problems in children (EFSA, 2009), estrogenic activity (Axon et al.), and potentially impact testicular health negatively (EFSA, 2009). Aluminum is neurotoxic (Inan-Eroglu) (Shaw et al.).

Hydrolyzed casein: difficult to digest, allergenic protein from milk linked to type 1 diabetes (Chia et al.). Anaphylaxis reactions to immunizations containing casein have been reported in the medical literature (Silva et al.).

Sucrose: table sugar (a disaccharide containing glucose and fructose).

D-sorbitol: sugar alcohol that occurs naturally but is also produced synthetically and is associated with gastrointestinal disturbances (Mäkinen et al.).

Formaldehyde: one of the most toxic substances known, a carcinogen (Swenberg et al.), corrosive (NJDH 2016), flammable gas (NJDH 2016), used in embalming fluid, is a byproduct of automotive exhaust, and is released from carpet and particle board. It is on the Right To Know Hazardous Substance List as cited by OSHA, ACGIH, DOT, NIOSH, NTP, DEP, IARC, IRIS, NFPA, and the EPA and is also on the Special Health Hazard Substance List. It causes cancer of the nasopharynx and leukemia (NJDH 2016).

Aluminum phosphate/hydroxide: toxic metal shown to cause osteomalacia, microcytic anemia, and encephalopathy/dementia (Willhite et al.). Aluminum is neurotoxic (Inan-Eroglu) (Shaw et al.) and may induce "oxidative stress, immunologic alterations, genotoxicity, pro-inflammatory effect, peptide denaturation or transformation, enzymatic dysfunction, metabolic derangement, amyloidogenesis, membrane perturbation, iron dyshomeostasis, apoptosis, necrosis and dysplasia" (Igbokwe et al.). Aluminum as a vaccine adjuvant can cause autoimmune diseases (Pellegrino et al.) (Dorea et al.) (Perricone et al.), chronic fatigue (Couette et al.), and cognitive dysfunction/deficits (Couette et al.) (Shaw et al.). Aluminum in vaccines can cause macrophagic myofasciitis, muscle weakness, MS symptoms, MS-like demyelinating disorders, etc. (Israeli et al.) (Authier et al.) (Gherardi et al.).

Trometamol: weakly toxic, biologically inert amino alcohol (Spadea et al.), a component of buffer solutions, increases cell membrane permeability. A gel form was associated with periorbital dermatitis (Spadea et al.).

Polysorbate 80 (Tween 80) (polyoxyethylene sorbitan mono-oleate): synthetic nonionic surfactant used widely as an additive in foods, pharmaceutical preparations, and cosmetics as an emulsifier, dispersant, or stabilizer (National Toxicology Program, 1992). Has been associated with an increased risk of systemic adverse events including hypersensitivity systemic reactions (Schwartzberg et al.), a number of reproductive problems in female rats (Gajdová et al.), hypotension and tachycardia in dogs (Millard et al.), and thrombocytopenia, pulmonary deterioration, ascites, and liver and renal failure, secondary to vasculopathic hepatotoxicity in pediatric patients (Kriegel et al.).

Neomycin sulfate: "broad spectrum aminoglycoside antibiotic derived from Streptomyces fradiae with antibacterial activity" (Pubchem). Causes nephrotoxicity and ototoxicity (Masur et al.).

Streptomycin: antibiotic shown to enhance the susceptibility to Salmonella infection (Bohnhoff et al.) and to enhance Candida growth (Campbell et al.).

Polymyxin B: Antibiotic. Neurotoxic and nephrotoxic (Falagas et al.).

Glutaraldehyde: low molecular weight aldehyde disinfectant. Side effects may include sensory irritant effects, sinus symptoms, and bronchitis (Takigawa), and potential neurotoxicity and developmental effects (Beauchamp et al.). Toxic to fish and birds (Leung et al.).

Host cell DNA benzonase: "genetically engineered endonuclease from Serratia marcescens". "Attacks and degrades all forms of DNA and RNA" (Millipore Sigma). Removes the nucleic acids from recombinant proteins by digesting DNA and RNA. Decreases the viscosity of protein extracts and prevents clumping of chimeric cell mixtures.

Deoxycholate: bile acid. Bile acid does not belong in your blood stream, it belongs in your gallbladder and duodenum.

Octoxynol-10 (TRITON X-100): poly(ethylene glycol) derivative non ionic surfactant. Acts as an emulsifier/detergent to solubilize proteins and permeabilizes living cell membranes (Koley et al.). In excess concentrations, it is fatal to human cells (Koley et al.). Strong evidence that it is a human skin toxicant or allergen (EWG Skin Deep Database).

Ammonium thiocyanate: on the hazardous substance list as cited by DOT and EPA, is a skin, eye, nose, and throat irritant (NJDH 2002), repeated exposure may cause headache, nausea, vomiting, loss of appetite, and weight loss (NJDH 2002), may affect the thyroid gland (NJDH 2002), may cause confusion, dizziness, convulsions, anxiety, and unconsciousness and death (NJDH 2002), harmful to aquatic life with long lasting effects (Labchem 2016), When handling this substance it is recommended to wear gloves, protective clothing, eye protection, and face protection (Fisher Science Education 2014).

Thimerosol: compound containing 49.6% ethyl mercury, a known neurotoxin and cardiotoxin that can cause over 250 symptoms (Dorea et al.) (Azevedo et al.) (Rice et al.). Over 89 peer reviewed articles have linked mercury, thimerosol, and autism (childrenshealthdefense.org). At least 180 studies have shown thimerosol to be harmful (Geier et al.). Six studies done by the CDC showing thimerosol in vaccines to be safe are unreliable and show evidence of scientific malfeasance (Hooker et al.). Boys who received hep B vaccines with mercury were 9 times more likely to become developmentally disabled versus unvaccinated boys (Gallagher et al.)

Live viruses: Many vaccines contain live viruses such as MMR, Varivax (varicella vaccine), Proquad, RotaTeq and Rotarix (rotavirus vaccines), Flu mist, Yellow fever vaccine, Adenovirus vaccine, Chickenpox vaccine, Typhoid vaccine, BCG, Smallpox vaccine, and the Oral Polio Vaccine. Natural measles and mumps infections (as opposed to ones caused by vaccination) in childhood are protective against fatal heart attacks and strokes during adulthood (Kubota et al.). Abnormal MMR antibody levels are found in children with autism and have been linked to MMR vaccination (Singh et al.). Young children are at an increased risk of requiring emergency care after MMR vaccination (Wilson et al.). Vaccinating children against chickenpox increases cases of fatal shingles in the elderly (Brisson et al.) (Luyten et al.) (Ogunjimi et al.). Acquiring chickenpox (varicella) naturally during childhood protects against coronary heart disease (Pesonen et al.) and the universal chickenpox vaccination program is not effective (Goldman et al.). The rotavirus vaccine, RotaTeq, may increase the risk of life-threatening intestinal damage and Kawasaki disease (Geier et al.). Polio vaccination in India probably caused thousands of children to be paralyzed (Vashisht et al.). Millions of people in the U.S. in the

1950's received a polio vaccine that was contaminated with the cancer causing SV40 virus due to being cultured in monkey kidneys (Shah et al.).

For more information:
https://www.cdc.gov/vaccines/pubs/pinkbook/downloads/appendices/b/excipient-table-2.pdf
http://www.vaccinesafety.edu/components-Excipients.htm
collingowcnc.wixsite.com/collingowcnc/articlesandprotocols

Post COVID-19 Vaccine Care

Collin Gow, C.N.C.

11/8/2021

It is important to know that many **side effects** have been reported by individuals after receiving COVID-19 "vaccinations". Anyone can report their adverse reactions to the **Vaccine Adverse Events Reporting System (VAERS)** at vaers.hhs.gov. VAERS is an early warning system that monitors vaccine safety in the U.S.. It is co-managed by the **FDA** and **CDC**. As of 10/22/21, **837,595 adverse events, including 17,619 deaths,** have been **reported** to VAERS after COVID-19 vaccination. The following table lists some of the current adverse events that have been reported to VAERS and the number of reports:

Guillain-Barre	1537
Acute Disseminated Encephalomyelitis	108
Transverse Myelitis	280
Encephalitis	1271
Convulsions/Seizures	10618
Stroke	9952
Narcolepsy, Cataplexy	200
Anaphylaxis	37281
Acute Myocardial Infarction (Heart Attack)	2840
Myocarditis/Pericarditis	9487
Autoimmune Disease	856
Other Acute Demyelinating Diseases	204
Pregnancy and birth outcomes (Miscarriages)	2526
Other Allergic Reactions	1601
Thrombocytopenia	3456
Disseminated Intravascular Coagulation	151
Venous Thromboembolism	15287
Arthritis and Arthralgia/Joint Pain	55097
Kawasaki Disease	32
Systemic Inflammatory Response Syndrome	473

The same **adverse event** outcomes have been listed by the **FDA** in their own documents also, which can be found here: https://www.fda.gov/media/143557/download. These are not all of the possible adverse reactions. There have been anecdotal reports of low white blood cell counts also.

The following is a screenshot of the **ingredients** in the **Pfizer, Moderna,** and **Johnson**

and Johnson vaccines, taken from Appendix C on cdc.gov:

Description	Pfizer-BioNTech (mRNA) For persons aged 5-11 years (10 µg dose) formulation	Pfizer-BioNTech (mRNA) For persons aged ≥12 years (30 µg dose) formulation	Moderna (mRNA) For persons aged ≥18 years	Janssen (viral vector) For persons aged ≥18 years
Active ingredient	Nucleoside-modified mRNA encoding the viral spike (S) glycoprotein of SARS-CoV-2	Nucleoside-modified mRNA encoding the viral spike (S) glycoprotein of SARS-CoV-2	Nucleoside-modified mRNA encoding the viral spike (S) glycoprotein of SARS-CoV-2	Recombinant, replication-incompetent Ad26 vector, encoding a stabilized variant of the SARS-CoV-2 Spike (S) protein
Inactive ingredients	2[(polyethylene glycol (PEG))-2000]-N,N-ditetradecylacetamide	2[(polyethylene glycol (PEG))-2000]-N,N-ditetradecylacetamide	PEG2000-DMG:1,2-dimyristoyl-rac-glycerol, methoxypolyethylene glycol	Polysorbate-80
	1,2-distearoyl-sn-glycero-3-phosphocholine	1,2-distearoyl-sn-glycero-3-phosphocholine	1,2-distearoyl-sn-glycero-3-phosphocholine	2-hydroxypropyl-β-cyclodextrin
	Cholesterol	Cholesterol	Cholesterol	Citric acid monohydrate
	(4-hydroxybutyl)azanediyl)bis(hexane-6,1-diyl)bis(2-hexyldecanoate)	(4-hydroxybutyl)azanediyl)bis(hexane-6,1-diylbis(2-hexyldecanoate)	SM-102:heptadecan-9-yl 8-((2-hydroxyethyl) (6-oxo-6-(undecyloxy) hexyl) amino) octanoate	Trisodium citrate dihydrate
	Tromethamine	Sodium chloride	Tromethamine	Sodium chloride
	Tromethamine hydrochloride	Monobasic potassium phosphate	Tromethamine hydrochloride	Ethanol
	Sucrose	Potassium chloride	Acetic acid	
		Dibasic sodium phosphate dihydrate	Sodium acetate	
		Sucrose	Sucrose	

A number of these ingredients are **synthetic** and may be harmful. In addition, it has been speculated by multiple doctors and researchers, upon examination under microscope, that some or all of these vaccines may possibly contain **graphene oxide** and other unknown materials not listed as ingredients. For more information on graphene oxide, go to https://odysee.com/@collingowcnc:7/GRAPHENE-OXIDE-NUTRACEUTICAL-ANTIDOTES-THE-BIOMOLECULAR-CORONA:a and watch the video depicted below:

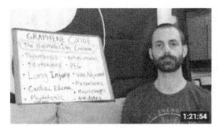

If you or a loved one is suffering from side effects from COVID-19 vaccination, there are remedies you or they may want to consider. **Pick 5 of the following:**

1. **Glutathione or NAC**, 500–1000mg 2x/day on empty stomach to detoxify harmful compounds
2. **Vital Earth Fulvic/Humic Mineral Blend or Shilajit** to detoxify graphene oxide
3. **Chaga**, 2–3g/day with food to boost S.O.D. (antioxidant enzyme), modulate immunity, protect DNA from damage, and repair DNA
4. **Cat's Claw**, 1000mg 2x/day with food to modulate immunity and protect the tissues and organs from damage and inflammation caused by the spike protein being produced in response to the vaccines
5. **Pine Needle Tea or Star Anise Tea**, (high in shikimic acid) 1–2 cups/day to reduce the damage and inflammation from the spike protein
6. **Ginger, Garlic, Fish Oil, Vitamin E, Nattokinase, Grapeseed Extract**, or very small amount of **Cayenne** to thin the blood and reduce clotting risk
7. **Zinc**, 15mg 2x/day and **Quercetin**, 1000mg 2x/day with food for immunity and allergy
8. **Vitamin D3**, 5,000–10,000 IU/day with food for immunity and allergy
9. **Fennel**, 1000mg 3x/day with meals to reduce damage and inflammation from the spike protein
10. **Curcumin**, 750mg 2x/day to reduce inflammation/cytokines
11. **Magnesium L-Threonate, St. John's Wort, Gotu Kola** (do not consume if pregnant), **Taurine, Choline, R-Lipoic Acid, Benfothiamine, Acetyl-L-Carnitine**, or a **Whole Food B-Complex** for nervous system protection, repair, and/or relaxation
12. **CoQ10, Pomegranate Juice, Hawthorn, Acetyl-L-Carnitine, Magnesium Taurate, Resveratrol, Garlic**, or **Red Wine Extract** for heart health/heart inflammation
13. **Vitamin K1** (ONLY IF THROMBOCYTOPENIA DEVELOPS AND ONLY IN COMBINATION WITH A REMEDY FROM #6 ON THIS LIST)

Eat a healthy diet containing high amounts of fruits, vegetables, herbs, spices, nuts, seeds, legumes, mushrooms, onions, garlic, seaweeds, **dark chocolate**, **tomatoes**, underground storage organs (potatoes, sweet potatoes, purple potatoes, yams, yuca, cassava), and squashes. Limit meats & processed foods. Minimal fish, egg yolks, & organ meats is okay (3oz/day).

Should I Vaccinate My Child for COVID-19 or Support My Child's Natural Immunity?

Collin Gow, C.N.C.

11/19/2021

About 40 doses of vaccines are already recommended by age 11 by the CDC on their immunization schedule. That information can be found here: https://www.cdc.gov/vaccines/schedules/hcp/imz/child-adolescent.html. Adding more "vaccines" to that schedule may not be the greatest idea, especially when you consider the ingredients in vaccines.

What are the ingredients in vaccines?

- Human fetal lung fibroblast cells
- Protein from human blood
- Monkey kidney cells
- Protein from cow blood
- Mutant of diptheria toxin
- Adhesive polymers
- Milk sugar
- Plasticizer chemicals (phthalates)
- Artificial dyes
- Acetone
- Aluminum
- Casein
- Mercury
- Sucrose
- Sugar alcohols
- Formaldehyde
- Amino alcohols
- Polysorbate 80
- Antibiotics
- Disinfectants
- Genetically engineered ingredients
- Bile acids
- Polyethylene glycol
- Ammonia
- Live viruses

https://www.cdc.gov/vaccines/pubs/pinkbook/downloads/appendices/b/excipient-table-2.pdf
http://www.vaccinesafety.edu/components-Excipients.htm

What are the ingredients in the Pfizer-Biontech COVID-19 "vaccine" for ages 5–11?
mRNA, lipids ((4-hydroxybutyl)azanediyl)bis(hexane-6,1-diyl)bis(2-hexyldecanoate), 2 [(polyethylene glycol)-2000]-N,N-ditetradecylacetamide, 1,2-Distearoyl-sn-glycero-3-phosphocholine, and cholesterol), tromethamine, tromethamine hydrochloride, sucrose, and sodium chloride.
https://www.fda.gov/media/153717/download

What side effects to COVID-19 vaccines have been reported?
Guillaine Barre, Acute Disseminated Encephalomyelitis, Transverse Myelitis, Encephalitis, Convulsions/Seizures, Stroke, Narcolepsy, Cataplexy, Anaphylaxis, Acute Myocardial Infarction (Heart Attack), Myocarditis/Pericarditis, Autoimmune Disease, Other Acute Demyelinating Diseases, Pregnancy and birth outcomes (Miscarriages), Other Allergic Reactions, Thrombocytopenia, Disseminated Intravascular Coagulation, Venous Thromboembolism, Arthritis and Arthralgia/Joint Pain, Kawasaki Disease, Systemic Inflammatory Response Syndrome, Death. vaers.hhs.gov
https://www.fda.gov/media/143557/download

Are vaccines safe and effective?
Considering the ingredients and side effects above, the answer has to be no, regardless of the fact that

some have undergone phase 1, 2, and 3 clinical trials (the Pfizer-Biontech "vaccine" has). At least half of the scientific literature in general these days may be untrue due to major conflicts of interest and other problems, (Gyles et al.). However, the CDC and other governing bodies claim that the COVID vaccines are safe and effective. But what does "safe and effective" actually mean? "Safe" means that a vaccine has undergone clinical trials, FDA review, and the benefits are said to outweigh the risks. "Effective" means that the vaccine has undergone clinical trials, been reviewed by the FDA, elicits an antibody response, and that it doesn't lose much effectiveness through storage and delivery.
https://www.cdc.gov/flu/vaccines-work/effectivenessqa.htm
https://www.cdc.gov/vaccinesafety/research/index.html
https://www.cdc.gov/vaccines/parents/infographics/journey-of-child-vaccine.html

What is the chance that my child will die of COVID-19?
There have been 94 COVID-19 deaths from January 1, 2020 to October 16, 2021 in children ages 5–11 in the U.S.. https://www.cdc.gov/vaccines/acip/meetings/downloads/slides-2021-11-2-3/03-COVID-Jefferson-508.pdf There were 24.4 million children aged 6-11 alive in the United States as of 2019.
https://www.statista.com/statistics/457786/number-of-children-in-the-us-by-age/
That is a 1 in 259,574 chance that a child between age 6-11 would die of COVID-19.

Can you sue a vaccine manufacturer if your child is damaged by a vaccine?
No. That is why the governmental National Vaccine Injury Compensation Program exists.

If your child has been injured by a vaccine and you are seeking compensation, go here:
https://www.hrsa.gov/vaccine-compensation/index.html
For COVID vaccine injury go here:
https://www.hrsa.gov/cicp

Is the Pfizer-Biontech COVID-19 vaccine FDA approved for children ages 5–11?
No. It has been authorized for emergency use only. It has not been FDA "approved". "Under an EUA [Emergency Use Authorization], FDA may allow the use of unapproved medical products, or unapproved uses of approved medical products in an emergency to diagnose, treat, or prevent serious or life-threatening diseases or conditions when certain statutory criteria have been met, including that there are no adequate, approved, and available alternatives. Taking into consideration input from the FDA, manufacturers decide whether and when to submit an EUA request to FDA."
https://www.fda.gov/news-events/press-announcements/fda-authorizes-pfizer-biontech-covid-19-vaccine-emergency-use-children-5-through-11-years-age

Has the Pfizer-Biontech COVID-19 vaccine been studied in children?
It has been studied for safety in approximately 3,100 children age 5 through 11 and "no serious side effects have been detected". Obviously, the FDA's definition of "side effects" is a pretty loose definition. "In addition, the vaccine was found to be 90.7% effective in preventing COVID-19 in children 5 through 11." https://www.fda.gov/news-events/press-announcements/fda-authorizes-pfizer-biontech-covid-19-vaccine-emergency-use-children-5-through-11-years-age

Can you trust the FDA, the CDC, and Pfizer?
The FDA receives 45% of its annual budget from the pharmaceutical industry. Bill Gates gave the CDC $1 million in 2003, $30 million in 2013/14, and he gave a combined $20 million to groups including the CDC in 2020 to combat COVID-19. This exorbitant private funding of a "public" agency creates conflicts of interest. Pfizer agreed to pay the largest criminal fine in U.S. history in 2009 at $2.3 billion

for fraudulent marketing. You tell me.

If my child gets "vaccinated" for COVID-19 can he or she still get COVID-19?
Yes. https://www.cdc.gov/coronavirus/2019-ncov/vaccines/effectiveness/why-measure-effectiveness/breakthrough-cases.html#:~:text=Most%20people%20who%20get%20COVID,%E2%80%9Cbreakthrough%20infection.%E2%80%9D

Why do we have an immune system?
To identify, neutralize, protect, and eliminate threats from other species or pathogenic microbes. The body has neutrophils, lymphocytes, monocytes, basophils, eosinophils, dendritic cells, macrophages, natural killer cells, mast cells, and other systems to deal with foreign invaders. Consider supporting your child's natural immunity for a robust antiviral response.

How Can I Support My Child's Natural Immunity?

Supplements
1. Baker's yeast or Nutritional Yeast or Beta-Glucans (Saccharomyces cerevisiae) have been shown to reduce the risk of respiratory infections in children, (Jesenak, Milos et al.)
2. Zinc, 5–10mg/day
3. Vitamin D3, 1,000–3,000IU/day
4. Probiotic, 1 Billion–5 Billion/day
5. Elderberry Syrup or Gummies
6. Lemon Balm Tincture
7. Echinacea/Astragalus Tincture
8. Multivitamin
9. Colostrum
10. Whole Food Vitamin C

Foods
Consume a healthy diet of whole fruits, vegetables, herbs, spices, underground storage organs (potatoes, sweet potatoes, purple potatoes), squashes, legumes, mushrooms, garlic, onions, ginger, peppers, citrus fruits, fermented foods, manuka honey, nutritional yeast, seaweed, pumpkin seeds, and brazil nuts. Limit refined and processed foods. Minimal amounts of fish, egg yolks, & organ meats is okay.

Post Virus Recovery

Collin Gow, C.N.C.

1/16/22

When a virus challenges your immune system, your body has to mount and carry out a defense against the attack. This is stressful on your body. It can deplete your reserves, dehydrate you, and cause inflammation. After fighting an infection, you may find yourself feeling fatigued, you may have lost your sense of taste or smell, your hair may be falling out, you may have a cough that won't go away, or you may have difficulty breathing, chest pain, muscle weakness, joint pain, headaches, brain fog, diarrhea, or other symptoms.[1-4] Your lungs, heart, brain, kidneys, and/or other systems may have been damaged. Histopathological findings could be endothelial damage, alveolar damage, pulmonary fibrosis, myocyte injury, hypoxic injury, tubular necrosis, glomerularsclerosis, or other issues.[4] You may be referred to as a "long-hauler" or someone may say that you have "post acute _____ syndrome". Certain drugs or supplements you took during illness may have given you after-effects as well. Fortunately, you can do something about it. Here are some natural food, supplement, and lifestyle considerations for each indication:

Fatigue and muscle weakness: multivitamin, carnitine, and olive leaf[5], rhodiola, schisandra, iron, COQ10, creatine, electrolytes, fruit, plant protein, calcium

Headaches, joint pain, chest pain: decaf green tea, resveratrol, cannabinoids, curcumin, and quercetin,[6] andrographis, devils claw, boswellia, msm, magnesium, arjuna, hawthorn, mung bean extract, omega-3s, olive leaf, carnitine

Dehydration: electrolyte, kelp, magnesium, hyaluronic acid, spring water, fruits and vegetables, bone broth

Hair loss/telogen effluvium: iron, vitamin C, and calories,[7] royal jelly, nettles, horsetail, collagen, bamboo extract

Loss of smell and taste (anosmia and aguesia): zinc,[8,9] smell training using rose, eucalyptus, lemon, and clove oils,[10] beta-caryophyllene,[10] raw honey, silver, vitamin A, echinacea, licorice tea, slippery elm lozenges, oral probiotic, & nerve remedies[10] such as lion's mane, choline, and a whole food b-complex

Brain fog: lion's mane, blue green algae, choline, serine, iodine, coconut oil, sage, berries

Chronic cough/lung damage/sensory neuropathic cough: EPA + GLA,[11] NAC, vitamin A, licorice, black seed oil, boswellia, silica, mullein, chickweed, horehound, coltsfoot, marshmallow, peppermint, eucalyptus, pleurisy, and nerve remedies[12] such as GABA, cannabinoids, taurine, lion's mane

Difficulty breathing: oxygen cans, iron, chlorophyll or copper, vitamin C, cordyceps, peppermint, carnitine, rhodiola, yohimbe, butcher's broom, Liquid Light, boswellia, mullein, chickweed, horehound, coltsfoot, marshmallow, licorice, pleurisy, NAC, Oxypower, vitamin A, citrus fruits, sea salt, spring water

Diarrhea: psyllium, prebiotic, probiotic, saccharomyces boulardii, red raspberry leaf, boswellia, vitamin A

Immune system support/other: cat's claw, fennel, pine needle tea, star anise, probiotic

All the above: Myers cocktail I.V.

Diet: eat a nearly plant-based diet,[13] with high amounts of fruits and vegetables, consume citrus, kelp, sea salt, plant protein, small amounts of liver (high in vitamin A), iron rich foods such as molasses, liver, kale, spinach, and legumes and drink spring water

Lifestyle: focus on sleep and rest before jumping back into your normal lifestyle and exercise routine. Reduce your work and stress load. Once all your symptoms are gone, choose low intensity, light forms of physical movement. Take a walk in nature. Practice qi gong or deep breathing exercises.

References:
1. Pavli A, Theodoridou M, Maltezou HC. Post-COVID Syndrome: Incidence, Clinical Spectrum, and Challenges for Primary Healthcare Professionals. Arch Med Res. 2021 Aug;52(6):575-581. doi: 10.1016/j.arcmed.2021.03.010. Epub 2021 May 4. PMID: 33962805; PMCID: PMC8093949.
2. Lopez-Leon S, Wegman-Ostrosky T, Perelman C, Sepulveda R, Rebolledo PA, Cuapio A, Villapol S. More than 50 long-term effects of COVID-19: a systematic review and meta-analysis. Sci Rep. 2021 Aug 9;11(1):16144. doi: 10.1038/s41598-021-95565-8. PMID: 34373540; PMCID: PMC8352980.
3. Cereda E, Clavé P, Collins PF, Holdoway A, Wischmeyer PE. Recovery Focused Nutritional Therapy across the Continuum of Care: Learning from COVID-19. Nutrients. 2021 Sep 21;13(9):3293. doi: 10.3390/nu13093293. PMID: 34579171; PMCID: PMC8472175.
4. Chippa V, Aleem A, Anjum F. Post Acute Coronavirus (COVID-19) Syndrome. [Updated 2021 Oct 1]. In: StatPearls [Internet]. Treasure Island (FL): StatPearls Publishing; 2021 Jan-. Available from: https://www.ncbi.nlm.nih.gov/books/NBK570608/
5. Naureen Z, Dautaj A, Nodari S, Fioretti F, Dhuli K, Anpilogov K, Lorusso L, Paolacci S, Michelini S, Guda T, Kallazi M, Bertelli M. Proposal of a food supplement for the management of post-COVID syndrome. Eur Rev Med Pharmacol Sci. 2021 Dec;25(1 Suppl):67-73. doi: 10.26355/eurrev_202112_27335. PMID: 34890036.
6. Giovinazzo G, Gerardi C, Uberti-Foppa C, Lopalco L. Can Natural Polyphenols Help in Reducing Cytokine Storm in COVID-19 Patients? Molecules. 2020 Dec 12;25(24):5888. doi: 10.3390/molecules25245888. PMID: 33322757; PMCID: PMC7763290.
7. Almohanna HM, Ahmed AA, Tsatalis JP, Tosti A. The Role of Vitamins and Minerals in Hair Loss: A Review. Dermatol Ther (Heidelb). 2019 Mar;9(1):51-70. doi: 10.1007/s13555-018-0278-6. Epub 2018 Dec 13. PMID: 30547302; PMCID: PMC6380979.
8. Propper RE. Smell/Taste alteration in COVID-19 may reflect zinc deficiency. J Clin Biochem Nutr. 2021 Jan;68(1):3. doi: 10.3164/jcbn.20-177. Epub 2021 Jan 1. PMID: 33536704; PMCID: PMC7844651.
9. Hummel T, Landis BN, Hüttenbrink KB. Smell and taste disorders. GMS Curr Top Otorhinolaryngol Head Neck Surg. 2011;10:Doc04. doi: 10.3205/cto000077. Epub 2012 Apr 26. PMID: 22558054; PMCID: PMC3341581.

10. Koyama S, Kondo K, Ueha R, Kashiwadani H, Heinbockel T. Possible Use of Phytochemicals for Recovery from COVID-19-Induced Anosmia and Ageusia. Int J Mol Sci. 2021 Aug 18;22(16):8912. doi: 10.3390/ijms22168912. PMID: 34445619; PMCID: PMC8396277.

11. Pacht ER, DeMichele SJ, Nelson JL, Hart J, Wennberg AK, Gadek JE. Enteral nutrition with eicosapentaenoic acid, gamma-linolenic acid, and antioxidants reduces alveolar inflammatory mediators and protein influx in patients with acute respiratory distress syndrome. Crit Care Med. 2003 Feb;31(2):491-500. doi: 10.1097/01.CCM.0000049952.96496.3E. PMID: 12576957.

12. Laryngopedia. (2021, March 3). *Still Coughing After COVID? | Sensory Neuropathic Cough (SNC)*. YouTube. Retrieved January 16, 2022, from https://www.youtube.com/watch?v=MWxbFiiQPi0

13. Storz MA. Lifestyle Adjustments in Long-COVID Management: Potential Benefits of Plant-Based Diets. Curr Nutr Rep. 2021 Dec;10(4):352-363. doi: 10.1007/s13668-021-00369-x. Epub 2021 Sep 10. PMID: 34506003; PMCID: PMC8429479.

Collin Gow, C.N.C.

is an author, certified nutritional consultant, naturevore,
naturotheologist, and father.

Collin's Websites

www.collingowcnc.wixsite.com/collingowcnc
www.collingowcnc.wixsite.com/naturevorenutrition
www.collingowcnc.wixsite.com/naturotheology
www.collingowcnc.com (under construction as of 1/25/2022)
www.naturevorenutrition.com (under construction as of 1/25/2022)
www.naturotheology.org (under construction as of 1/25/2022)

Collin's Other Books

- *Collin Gow, C.N.C.: Collected Works on Health and Nutrition, Volume 1 (2017–2020)*

- *The Night Before Winter Solstice: An Earth and Nature-Based Spin on a Christmas Classic*

- *Collin Gow, C.N.C.: An Anthology of Artworks (2004–2020)*

- *Collin Gow, C.N.C.: Collected Works on Health and Nutrition, Volume 2 (2021–2022)*

All available for purchase on Amazon @
https://www.amazon.com/Collin-Gow-C.N.C./e/B08RWMRYQR
%3Fref=dbs_a_mng_rwt_scns_share

Made in the USA
Las Vegas, NV
02 May 2024

89403693R00033